T0271640

SICK OF IT

Sophie Harman

SICK OF IT

The Global Fight for Women's Health

virago

VIRAGO

First published in Great Britain in 2024 by Virago Press

1 3 5 7 9 10 8 6 4 2

Copyright © Sophie Harman 2024

The moral right of the author has been asserted.

A CIP catalogue record for this book
is available from the British Library.

Hardback ISBN 978-0-349-01720-4
Trade Paperback ISBN 978-0-349-01721-1

Typeset in Sabon by M Rules
Printed and bound in Great Britain by
Clays Ltd, Elcograf S.p.A.

Papers used by Virago are from well-managed forests
and other responsible sources.

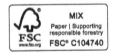

Virago Press
An imprint of
Little, Brown Book Group
Carmelite House
50 Victoria Embankment
London EC4Y 0DZ

An Hachette UK Company
www.hachette.co.uk

www.virago.co.uk

For Peris

Contents

PART 3:
SOS! (SAME OLD SOLUTIONS)

Introduction

There Has Never Been a Constitutional Crisis Over a Prostate

The point at which I really became sick of it was in February 2020. It happened when I walked into the Ministry of Health in downtown Freetown, Sierra Leone and someone checked my temperature and asked me to wash my hands. It was the sinking feeling that it was going to happen again.

For two weeks up to that point, I had been in Freetown talking to women about the impact of Ebola on their lives during the 2014/16 outbreak. I was on research leave from my usual day job as a professor teaching global health politics at a London university, and was in the country to investigate how health emergencies impact on women's lives. Over two weeks in Freetown, women told me how they had to improvise their own PPE (personal protective equipment) as they went about their front-line healthcare work, how more women died of pregnancy- and birth-related complications than Ebola itself, and how rates of domestic violence had increased because of stay-at-home orders. Women explained to me that they had been exhausted by keeping their family and friends sane during the crisis while doing wider work to help their friends and neighbours in the community. Many were outraged when girls who had become pregnant during Ebola were banned from returning to school when they reopened in April 2015. I learned how the outbreak had completely disrupted major aid programmes trying to end Sierra Leone's reputation for being one of the worst places in the world to be pregnant and give birth. And how a health system already struggling to deal with a brain drain of health workers moving abroad to find better-paid work depended on unpaid women to fill the gaps. Women told me how they were crying out for the international community to help mitigate the impact of the Ebola crisis on women and their health, but no one would listen unless they had good data proving something was afoot. And how once they got the data, no one believed them. As I washed my hands that day, the World Health Organization had put the world on warning about another major health emergency, COVID-19. I knew that everything the women in Freetown had told me risked happening again to other women. I felt sick at the inevitability that, should the COVID-19 health emergency get worse, it would be women who bore the brunt.

By February 2020, I had spent fifteen years researching global health politics, looking at how major diseases and foreign aid funding impact on women and their lives. As a professor of international politics, I had conducted research all over the world and sat in meetings with governments, donors, militaries, NGOs, community groups, activists and other academics, listening, discussing and advising on how to make sense of global health threats. I had spent time tracing how decisions made in Washington, New York and Geneva translate to national health ministries and rural healthcare settings, often with little understanding of how healthcare works in these parts of the world. I had made a film with women living with HIV/AIDS in Tanzania to try and get people to notice them. Most politicians and international organisations rarely considered the impact of health emergencies on women until it was too late, and women's bodies have always been a site of contested politics. I thought I'd wrap up the project in Sierra Leone, write some academic papers and move onto something else.

But that day in Freetown was a wake-up call. It was not just the coming threat of COVID-19 to women's lives – as massive as I knew that was going to be – but a nagging sense that progress on women's health was going backwards. Donald Trump had been president for three years and was wreaking havoc on women's health by cutting funding to family planning programmes in the US and abroad. Around the world populist politicians were uniting around the need to curtail women's access to reproductive health care, with dire consequences for women's health and well-being. A decade of austerity in Europe was changing how governments thought about foreign aid funding to women's health in poor countries. Maternity hospitals had become targets in war zones. Health inequalities for women persisted between rich countries in the global north and poorer countries in the global south. And then there were persistent inequalities within countries. In the UK, where I live, for example, a landmark study had been published two years earlier, presenting clear data that black women were five times more likely to die from pregnancy and childbirth complications than white women.

On top of all of this it seemed to me that the very organisations in the world responsible for advancing women's health were part of the problem. Scandals were emerging about the UN's involvement in sexual abuse and exploitation of women and girls in an Ebola outbreak in the Congo. The solution to these problems seemed to rest on getting women to sort it all out. Post #MeToo, lots of people in power started talking about gender equality in healthcare and male bias in science, but all this seemed to add up to was counting the women who sat on panels, authored publications and participated in clinical trials.

I knew I was not alone in thinking that the world seemed seriously scary and messed up for women, and that the different attacks and neglect of our health were somehow connected. I wanted to work out what connected all this turbulence. If another pandemic was to come along, would women, yet again, end up as substitute teachers/carers/unprotected health workers/victims of domestic abuse? Why did it feel like things were going backwards after twenty years of unprecedented investment in women's health? And what about all the preventable causes of death? Why is AIDS still the leading cause of death of young women, with one woman becoming infected with HIV every minute? And why will one woman die in the next two minutes from preventable complications linked to pregnancy and childbirth? The question I kept coming back to was simple: why do women still die when they don't have to?

As I started to think about my nagging questions, I realised the thread that connected all the turbulence was how central women's health is to how global politics works. Not just in the most obvious way – through reproduction being the backbone of economies, or politicians controlling women's bodies through abortion – or just in health emergencies and pandemics. But also in surprising and unpredictable ways, from some countries using successes in women's health as part of their diplomatic branding, to champions of gender equality doing everything in their power to block women leading international health agencies. Some of the worst offenders in abusing women's health for political gain aren't your usual right-wing politicians, but the very people who are supposed to be helping improve women's health. There were two sides to the problem – how women's health is exploited as a political issue, and how women themselves are exploited in the health sector.

Women's health is huge currency in global politics. If you want to get elected, forge diplomatic relations, change the politics and society of another country, gain international recognition in the world or make money for your charity, one of the best political tools with which to do so is women's health. In turn, if you want to run a health system, a major health campaign or project, or sustain a million-dollar aid budget, you need women's cheap, or sometimes free, labour and expertise. The world works off the back of exploiting women's health, but rarely for the purposes of improving women's health. This is why nothing changes for the better.

It's a total misconception to suggest women's health gets little attention in the world or political leaders don't really care about it. Far from it. Some aspects of women's health – notably reducing the number of women dying from childbirth- and pregnancy-related complications – are the number-one thing that governments around the world continuously agree to act on. This has led to countless global strategies, billions of aid dollars and high-profile proclamations at the UN, all centred on women's health. Women's health has visibility, money, prominent women leaders calling for change, global political commitments, a women-majority workforce, the knowledge to stop preventable death, and strategies and targets to make prevention a reality. Women's health gets loads of attention. It's just the wrong kind. This attention never has the purpose of making women healthier and happier. Gosh, no. Women's health either gets too much attention for the wrong reasons – trying to curtail women's access to contraception, winning votes by keeping the 'tradition' of FGM (female genital mutilation) or restricting abortion – or not enough attention for the right reasons – research, funding, correcting male bias in science.

Women die when they don't have to, not because of a lack of attention, science or evidence on what works for women's

health, but because of the exploitation of women's health
as a means of attaining and sustaining power in the world.
This book is the starting point to stopping this sick politics:
explaining how using and abusing women's health for political ends works and how it stops us making real strides in
women's health. It does not offer quick-fix easy solutions to
these problems. If anything, it strongly argues against such
quick fixes, which just add to an endless feedback loop of add
more women, then a different woman, to structures that fail
women. I'm not going to leave you without answers, though:
there are clear suggestions at the end of the book as to what
you can to do cope, resist and enact change. And the book
points to stories and evidence of women from across the
world coming together towards progress, as they have done
for centuries. They are the ones who are already calling out
politicians in their national governments and the international
organisations that shape so much of women's health. It is these
women whom this book is inspired by and dedicated to.

But what about men? You know men are dying, too?
    Whenever I talk about women's health, I get asked one of
these questions. When these questions fail to provoke a reaction in me, people ask me which women I am talking about,
as if I don't know women are hugely diverse, with differing
intersecting inequalities and advantages, interests, needs and
politics. Before we get going, allow me to clear two things
up so there are no unnecessary distractions and, selfishly, so
that no one asks me the man question ever again (although I
bet they still will). First, throughout the book I use the term
woman or women to refer to *all* women, and only specify
particular categories of women (which are also hugely diverse) – rich, poor, white, black, trans, of colour, living with
disability, living in a specific country or region of the world,
for example – when necessary to recognise the difference

in their health experiences, outcomes and types of political exploitation. There is more that unites women in how our health is exploited in global politics than divides us. Second, this is not a book that centres on men and men's health, and for good reason.

Men and boys also die of preventable causes. Gendered norms around what it is to be a man screw men and their health. Expectations that men and boys should be masculine and strong, and not talk about their feelings, impact on the health of billions of men around the world. Masculinity can be a barrier to men seeking out support and treatment that could help them lead happier and healthier lives. It prevents men from opening up about how they are feeling and discussing serious mental health issues such as depression. According to the leading health authority in the world, the WHO, men make up the vast majority of global death by suicide cases. In the UK, suicide is the biggest killer of men under forty-five. In the US, Argentina and Russia, men are four times more likely than women to die by suicide.

Men are also less likely than women to go to the doctor to seek help for physical and mental health problems, which has a knock-on impact on women and girls who have to suffer the impact of their behaviour when they don't get help and who have to seek out health facilities and medicines on behalf of their husbands, brothers, boyfriends, uncles, grandparents etc. But back to men ...

The questions that people ask me about men's health are rarely asked in pursuit of improving men's health and challenging the gender stereotypes that produce all kinds of inequality in health. The questions are a political act to silence women and limit the importance of discussing women's health or correcting male bias within science. Trying to shut me up and centre men or distract from a focus on women is part of a wider pattern of how power is embedded in women's health, of how women's health is diminished or framed as unexceptional. Anyone who questions this is silenced. It overlooks one of the fundamental problems of women's health: women's health is exceptional compared to men's because of how it is used as a political tool around the world.

There has never been a constitutional crisis over a prostate. Governments and courts don't argue about a country's constitution off the back of men wanting to have a vasectomy. States don't show off about how they have improved treatment and survival rates of prostate cancer as a means of demonstrating to the world how advanced they are. Presidents do not cover up political murders by citing high rates of vaccination of men and boys. It is not men in poor countries who are told to have fewer children as the (wrong) solution to climate change. When the international community wants to end poverty, they don't get men to do the donkey work. Men expect to be paid for the work they do in health settings, and are rarely expected to volunteer to care for family and neighbours as an act of love. When men work in health, they are seen as leaders and tend to be appointed to more senior and better paid positions. When men lead organisations it is the norm; when women do so they get held to a higher standard, and it is assumed they will represent every interest of every woman in the world. Women are left to die for routine reasons. And, let's face it, if men gave birth, they would not have to do so in car parks, at army checkpoints or without help or pain relief. When abortion is banned, it is other women collectively organising, driving other women across state borders to access healthcare and ordering abortion pills from the internet. It is not men. With the notable exception of the early AIDS crisis, the only time people ever get cross about men's health is when men give birth. Otherwise men and their health are left alone. Men take for granted that their health matters.

*

Women are sick of their health being used by politicians when it suits them and then forgotten about when help is needed. We are sick of men asking us what about them and their health when the whole world is organised around their needs and their right to be ignored. We are sick of it because we know it doesn't have to be this way.

In three parts, I am going to explain how the exploitation of women's health in global politics works, why it is the reason women die when they don't have to, and what you can do about it. The first part of the book, 'Saving Mothers', looks at how women's health – specifically maternal healthcare – is used as a tool to gain and sustain power in the world. The second part, 'Exploiting Women', concentrates on the way women are exploited within health and foreign aid sectors, often as collateral damage in the wider delivery of healthcare. The women featured in this section vary from underpaid community health workers to young women and girls exploited, abused and harassed by male health workers. The third part of the book looks at some of the same old solutions – 'SOS!' – we are always told will help women's health: leadership, gender experts, better data. It explains how these solutions can fail in practice, and what can be done about them. The final chapter in the book is one of hope and persistence, of women delivering change in health for other women. If you're up for challenging this sick politics of exploiting women's health for political gain, and for stopping women from dying when they don't have to, the Epilogue will show you how: from the easy things you can do to the bigger stuff that takes a bit more effort but is worth it.

I don't want you ever to feel like I did in February 2020, knowing how bad something can be and feeling you can't do anything about it. Thinking that the attacks on women's health are so big and overwhelming that you don't even know where to start with fighting back. Such feelings rob us of our collective power. I wrote this book to make you feel less alone and disempowered when it comes to women's health around the world, and to help you understand how global politics works to exploit women's health as a means of changing it.

Part 1

Saving Mothers

1

Soft Power and Healthwashing

In 1994, Rwanda was devastated by a genocide in which approximately 800,000 people were killed, many by their friends and neighbours, in a matter of days. In the aftermath, Rwanda's health and health system, like the rest of the country's soul and infrastructure, were on its knees. Post-genocide, Rwandans had the lowest life expectancy and highest rate of child mortality in the world. Ninety-four per cent of health workers had either been killed or had fled the country during the genocide, and many healthcare facilities and supply chains had been destroyed by the conflict.[1] Rwanda did not have any trauma surgeons or psychiatrists.[2] By the end of 1994, months after the genocide had ended, Rwanda was receiving some of the lowest contributions of foreign aid compared to other African countries, and was limited in terms of what it could borrow as a designated low-income country in international credit markets.[3] There was the persistent threat of HIV/AIDS, malaria and tuberculosis. The outlook for Rwanda's health, as with many post-conflict countries, was bleak. If health in the country continued to decline, even more people would die from preventable causes than had during the genocide.

The story of what happened next is extraordinary. Rwanda

made the health of the country a priority, and put women and their health at the centre of this. Between 2000 and 2015, following the genocide, Rwanda's investment in health translated into incredible results: under-five child mortality decreased by 70 per cent; there was a rapid decline in deaths from two of the biggest killers on the continent – malaria and AIDS; 97 per cent of children were vaccinated for ten key diseases (a higher vaccination rate than the US); 45.1 per cent of eligible women had access to modern contraception; it launched the first cancer treatment centre in rural Africa; 69 per cent of births in the country were attended by skilled birth attendants; and there was an astonishing 85 per cent reduction in maternal mortality.[4] The country met the UN standard of 80 per cent of people living with HIV being on life-saving treatment, and made sure women who contracted HIV on account of sexual violence during the war were first in the queue. The genocide undoubtedly played a role in prioritising the needs of survivors of sexual violence, but as a report in the medical journal the *Lancet* stated, 'The equity agenda was explicit' in Rwanda's health revolution.[5] Post-genocide, the leaders of the country wanted to rebuild in a way that recognised the contributions and needs of women in society. Rwanda therefore not only prioritised the international targets on women's health, it also transcended these to think through the relationship between rape as a weapon of war and women's health. Later, Rwanda was one of the first African countries to immunise girls against HPV – human papillomavirus. The leaders of Rwanda believed that women in poor, post-conflict countries deserved the same advanced cancer services as women in rich countries.

Such impressive results would be incredible for any country to achieve, even more so for a low- to middle-income country emerging from conflict and genocide. Rwanda also showed that a poor country could invest in health and deliver better health outcomes for women while growing its economy.

Between 2002 and 2012, Rwanda reported annual growth rates of 8 per cent, took one million people in the population out of poverty, and was ranked by the World Bank as the third most business-friendly destination in Africa.[6] Health and, more importantly, women's health, was not an afterthought but central to the future and growth of the country. Rwanda became *the* model of what happens to women's health when a government chooses to prioritise it. Such prioritisation was not without political motive. Women's health was about improving both the lives of women and the reputation of the Rwandan government.

In the aftermath of the genocide, the government of Rwanda knew no one else was coming to rebuild its health system. The international community's failure to call the genocide what it was and act to prevent or stop it gave a clear signal to Rwanda's politicians that if you want to change your country, you can't wait for others to help you. Change would be led by Rwandans for Rwanda, not by foreign aid agencies and consultants that appear in countries after a conflict with their own ideas and priorities. As Jean Pierre Nyemazi, a senior member of the Rwandan Ministry of Health who advises the WHO, put it, 'Countries really need to sit and understand the issues they faced themselves first, instead of throwing the responsibility to external donors or technical assistants.'[7] To sit and understand the issues, Rwanda took what is called a 'burden and gap approach' – it looked at where the major burdens and gaps in health were and who they were impacting upon the most.[8] Unsurprisingly, as with many health sectors in low-income countries, the burden of poor health was falling on women both in regard to their own health and well-being and their caring responsibilities for others, and the gaps were in primary healthcare and prevention, notably with regard to maternal mortality. To address the burden and gap and transform the health system, the Rwandan government would have to prioritise women's health.

Making women's health a priority was not just about the burdens and gaps in the health system. It was also about who was in charge and, crucially, Rwanda's commitment to gender parity across its political structures post the 1994 genocide. Rwanda's 2003 constitution states women should make up at least 30 per cent of all decision-making bodies in government. This is engineered at the national level, through twenty-four seats in the legislature being reserved for women. In 2008, Rwanda became the first parliament in the world to have a female majority and ten years after the passing of the new constitution, in 2013, women made up 64 per cent of parliamentary seats in the country. Women parliamentarians have reformed numerous policies to improve gender equality, including equal access and ownership of land, succession and inheritance rights, pay and labour laws, measures to end gender-based violence and, of course, they have made women's health a political priority within the country.[9] Add presidential commitment from Rwanda's leader, Paul Kagame, and Rwanda's health sector had the clear backing of the government to create change.

Driving this change was one dynamic woman leader, described by the *Lancet* as 'her government's greatest asset' and the BBC as 'one of the most important public health figures in the world today, if not the most important, and who has led some of the most remarkable declines in premature mortality the world has ever seen': Agnes Binagwaho.[10] Binagwaho had previously worked within the Rwandan health sector as the executive secretary of Rwanda's National AIDS Control Commission, permanent secretary of the Ministry of Health, and then minister of health for five years. When President Kagame asked her to take on transforming the health sector, her first instinct was to decline, given the scale of the challenge.[11] Like a lot of Rwandans, she had had been living in France during the genocide. But she knew if Rwandans like her didn't go back and fix the problem, no one would. So, she did.

As soon as Binagwaho took on the role, she was given a clear instruction by Kagame: 'Don't come here to do Politics. We want results.'[12] Tying future funding to clearly defined results can be a highly effective tool in advancing women's health, as it not only shows where progress is being made, but also where a health system or facility is failing, neglecting or not delivering for women and their health. If you combine this knowledge with government commitment to women's health, you can pinpoint where to put more or less money and/or political pressure to improve results for women. Rwanda did this with great success through what is called performance- or results-based financing – PBF or RBF for short. The idea is you create a set of targets and indicators and when health clinics hit these targets they receive more money. Money for performance or results – i.e. hitting the targets – is meant to motivate the health sector and individuals within it to do even better. This should be a win-win, because it motivates health professionals and ensures money keeps flowing to much-needed health issues for women. Health professionals don't have to worry about the money stopping as they know it will keep flowing if they perform and commit to women's health. Donors and health ministries can track where their money is going and therefore worry less about corruption. Women are part of the incentive structure, with health clinics incentivising women to come and give birth alongside skilled birth attendants (super important to improving mum and baby survival). Everyone wins.

Results are all very well from the supply side of health where you provide fully staffed and equipped health facilities, but to deliver better outcomes for women's health you also need to make sure women can access and afford quality care. Doing this in Rwanda meant providing health services and access within communities. Community health provision is important for everyone, but it is particularly important for women. Women living in poor rural communities – though really this applies to all women – have greater burdens on their time as they almost always have to engage in paid work, do the vast proportion of unpaid labour in the home and take on additional care burdens for their families and communities. Hence, women have less time to travel long distances outside their communities to access healthcare, may not be able to do so without the permission of a man, will put the health and needs of everyone else before their own and so defer travel for health until they really need to, by which point it is often too late. Centring health workers and services in the communities in which women live cuts the additional time burden for women and responds to their specific needs. Rwanda knew this and developed interventions that would help target these needs by introducing a system that connected community health workers to central health authorities, and ensured health was affordable and accessible to all through a community-based insurance scheme, the *mutuelle de santé*.[13]

Many countries have tried similar policies on women's health – particularly on maternal mortality – with mixed or little progress. Rwanda was different as it hit on a magic formula: focus on results + affordable, community-based healthcare + an effective woman leader in the health sector who has the backing of women parliamentarians and the president = better health outcomes for women. The story of Rwanda shows that if you look at where the burdens and gaps lie in the health sector, women's health will become a priority. And that when you make women's health a priority you can deliver results. If you can deliver better health for women in a poor, post-conflict country like Rwanda, you can do it anywhere. This is definitely the story that the government of Rwanda wants to put out into the world, but it is only part of the story.

The transformation of women's health in Rwanda came at a time when the international community was looking for a success story. As the next chapter shows in more detail, the late 1990s and early 2000s were a pivotal moment in women's health. One of the few issues world leaders could agree on during this time was the need to reduce maternal mortality, particularly in low- and middle-income countries and the continent with the highest rates of maternal death, Africa. The UN and major aid agencies were doing everything in their power to get other countries to do the same as Rwanda. The problem was that as much as countries claimed maternal health was a priority, results on improving the number of deaths from childbirth were not appearing as fast as hoped. For poor African countries, Rwanda became the model of what they should do to improve women's health – if a country like Rwanda could do it, so could they – and for aid donors, Rwanda showed that investment in women's health worked. Follow the Rwanda method and the international community could deliver a *global* success story on women's health.

Rwanda became a donor darling. So called because donors loved what the country was doing for women's health and continued to pour money into the country to support its efforts. This boosted the reputation of the country in both the medical science and aid communities, attracting new partners and opening up investment and diplomatic opportunities. Contrary to the story the Rwandan government likes to tell – that Rwanda transformed its health sector alone – at its peak in 2009, foreign aid made up 67 per cent of the country's health spending.[14] Rwanda has the highest aid per capita in East Africa.[15] All of the major health donors in the world – the

US, the EU, the Bill & Melinda Gates Foundation, the Global
Fund to Fight AIDS, Tuberculosis and Malaria, and the World
Bank – all have a strong presence in the country.

To top it all off, in 2014, Rwanda, in partnership with three
international partners – the Bill & Melinda Gates Foundation,
the Cummings Foundation and Partners In Health – created
a university dedicated to levelling up inequities in health:
the University of Global Health Equity. Women's health
and gender equality is central to the university's brand: it
has a specialist programme on gender, sexual and reproductive health delivery, a commitment to ensuring 70 per cent
of the intake for its flagship MSc in global health delivery
is made up of women, and a mentorship programme for
women and gender equality in science, medicine and global
health through its specialist Centre for Gender Equity.[16] All
of which is perhaps unsurprising given Agnes Binagwaho –
Rwanda's transformational health minister – served as one
of the first vice-chancellors of the university. The university
builds Rwanda's reputation and esteem in the world not just
by what it does on women's health, but who it partners: Bill
Gates, one of the richest men in the world and major health
philanthropist, and Paul Farmer of Partners In Health, a
hugely respected doctor and global advocate on the right of
the poor to access healthcare.

International recognition for Rwanda's overall health success
snowballed. The Rwandan health model has become the subject
of research in leading science and medical journals. Rwandan
health experts have an international profile in health diplomacy
through UN positions and international advisory boards. The
international community flocks to Rwanda's state-of-the-art
conference facilities, with major women's health conferences
taking place there. One such is Women Deliver, a global organisation that 'champions gender equality and the health and
rights of girls and women, in all their intersecting identities'[17],

who held their annual conference in the country in 2019 and 2023. When the African Union launched its ambitious strategy to transform vaccine manufacturing on the continent – to increase production of all vaccines used by the continent from 1 per cent made in Africa to 60 per cent by 2040 – it did so in Rwanda, with Kagame announcing the New Public Health Order, putting Africa at the centre of global health security. By 2023, to fully understand how women's health worked in the world you had to pass through one, if not all three, major hubs of power in global health: Geneva and Washington – where the main global health and international aid agencies are based – and Kigali, Rwanda's capital.

In the past, Rwanda's position in the world was defined by the 1994 genocide. Now, Rwanda uses women's health to define its reputation, status and influence in the world. Rwanda is a pioneer not only in its successful health outcomes for women, but also in using women's health as a tool of soft power. It uses success stories in women's health to gain global recognition and legitimacy with some of the most powerful states and philanthropists in the world, keep aid flowing to the country, build future education, research and knowledge, and to use such recognition to cement the country's position as one of the major powers within Africa. In turn, access to this sort of aid and diplomatic standing compounds the image of Rwanda as a major player in Africa and the world.

Using women's health as a tool of soft power is not necessarily a bad thing: it would be great if all the countries in the world gained their standing, recognition and good diplomacy from helping women. But there is a sinister side to this. Rwanda uses its standing on women's health to 'healthwash' the unseemly, more murderous part of Rwandan politics.

In theory, Rwanda is a presidential republic with a multiparty democracy and a tripartite division of power between the executive of the president and Cabinet; legislature of the Chamber of Deputies and Senate; and judiciary. Representatives that sit in the Chamber of Deputies are elected through proportional representation, and the president is elected by direct popular vote. As outlined above, Rwanda ticks all the right gender equality boxes: not only does it prioritise women's health, it was the first country in the world to have a female majority in parliament. On paper, then, Rwanda is a progressive democracy, leading the way in women's representation and gender equality policies.

The reality is quite different. Since the genocide in 1994, Rwanda has been ruled by one party – the Rwandan Patriotic Front (RPF) – and one man, Paul Kagame. Kagame officially became president in 2000, but had considerable influence on the government in the late 1990s. Since becoming president, Kagame has changed the constitution, which previously restricted the leader to two terms only, to allow him to run for three and then four terms. When Kagame ran for president in 2003, 2010 and 2017, he received approximately 90 per cent of the vote each time. This is not a marker of his popularity: any election observer (unless they work for an authoritarian regime) will tell you it is impossible for any leader to receive such a high percentage of the vote. The government of Rwanda has waged a sustained campaign of political repression against opposition parties. Any critics of the government are called out as partaking in 'divisive ideology'. Opposition politicians have been arrested, imprisoned or disappeared. Foreign media, such as the BBC, have been suspended from the country for periods of time, for speaking out on issues such as election results, the suspicious deaths of journalists or anything that questions the government's official position on the genocide, which the government would rather were kept quiet.[18]

Rwanda is reportedly a political regime that murders

ex-friends, opponents *and* allies, loots from neighbouring states, spies on citizens and visitors via their phones and laptops, prolongs civil wars in countries such as the Democratic Republic of Congo (DRC) and Burundi, and silences opposition.[19] According to journalist Michela Wrong, none of this is a secret. Those complicit in these crimes have admitted it. As Wrong clearly breaks down in her book *Do Not Disturb*, Kagame has been filmed 'effectively boasting' about the murder of ex-RPF politician Seth Sendashonga.[20] The UN has investigated and reported on the looting of the DRC.[21] A magistrate court in South Africa found the Rwandan government guilty of the murder of Kagame's comrade-in-arms and ex-head of Intelligence, Patrick Karegeya, and that the Rwandan government had put pressure on the government of South Africa to cover it up. Rwandan exiles in Sweden and the UK have been informed about threats to their life by the national security services.

Murderous authoritarian regime is not the reputation Rwanda wants in the world. This is where women's health comes in. Healthwashing works in two ways: deflection and complicity. Deflection is the easy bit. Saving mothers from dying is the ultimate 'yes, but' deflection tool. As we will see time and again in this book, women's health, particularly the notion of saving mothers, has strong political currency in the world: it is an issue that no one can disagree with, or wants to undermine efforts towards, and is an incredibly useful tool for politicians to use to justify a range of measures, from abortion bans to war to political disappearances. If you combine this with delivering a feminist women's health utopia – women-led health reforms, positive discrimination to train up women scientists and doctors of the future, and a health system that is designed around how women use it – you have a compelling counter story that shows you are a country that not only gets good health outcomes, but is also progressive and committed to social and gender justice to boot. Yes, there have been some political disagreements, but look at the HPV vaccination rates; yes, there are some disappearances, but look at how we prioritised women in our AIDS response.

For deflection to work, you need complicity. Scientists, medics, women's health advocates and world leaders who endorse and promote the success story of Rwanda are what make healthwashing work. Advocates who would usually oppose human-rights abuses instead defend and legitimise the offending state. People involved with the Rwandan health sector face a difficult choice: support a state that has seen tremendous advancements in health, particularly for women, or call out the other side of the story and diminish the state's reputation and thus the external funding that has supported such advancements. This is not a straightforward choice. They may be too reliant on the health sector for their livelihood/ degree/promotion to call out what is happening. In extreme cases, they could be too scared.

What in effect often happens with healthwashing is a slow complicity. Working in the Rwandan health sector gives people a sense of pride at what has been and what might yet be achieved. If you put long hours into achieving incredible results, it is an insult to suggest this effort is for some purpose other than simply improving the lives of Rwandans. Some people may play politics with what you achieve, but this is not why you do the work. International partners maintain a cognitive dissonance between Rwanda's health and Rwanda's politics as a means to continue to support the country. And you can see why. As the other chapters in this book will show, advances in women's health are so difficult that you have to celebrate the wins. A Rwandan government official would probably respond to this chapter by saying their politics is Rwanda's business, the country has shown incredible success, and if you don't like it, keep your nose out and don't make trouble. Besides, name a country that doesn't have a problematic history of political violence; it is unfair to pick on Rwanda.

If you think authoritarian rule is a good way of getting successful health results or is something you can turn a blind eye to, then I advise caution. Authoritarian rulers can ration who does or does not get access to health, rule the health sector by fear not trust (which has long-term implications for people working in the health sector and seeking out care) and create power vacuums when they leave power (whenever that may be). Light tolerance of authoritarian rule by international partners is fine while the country gets results, but as soon as the results stop and the authoritarian is seen to overstep the mark, the international community will turn their back on them. Zimbabwe is a cautionary tale: a country with one of the best health systems in Africa under the early years of Robert Mugabe's rule, which was ruined by the time of his death by the dual impact of authoritarianism and isolation from the international community. Women and women's health certainly do not benefit from increased isolation and growing authoritarianism: their health needs are often the first to be reversed. Kagame will definitely have one eye on Rwanda not becoming another Zimbabwe, but ultimately political actions of authoritarian rulers will come home to roost for the health sector. Fundamentally, the lives of women who have benefited from and been saved by Rwanda's health sector should not have more value than the lives of political opponents to Kagame.

Fundamentally, the means/ends argument demonstrates the power and efficacy of using women's health to wash the reputation and politics of Rwanda. It feels impolite to bring up Rwanda's acts of political murder or repression in health circles, as if I am the party pooper who has ruined a celebration of women's health and the achievements of a dedicated group of people working in extraordinary circumstances. We want to be able to disassociate the two. But we can't do this when domestic and international health leaders are the ones doing the washing. Healthwashing human-rights abuses and authoritarianism is a clear example of how women's health is used as a political tool. Rwanda exploits success in women's health to deflect negative attention and extend its influence and reputation in global politics. This is not just a stain on the reputation of Rwanda, but on all of the aid and global-health sector that validates prioritising women's health goals over blatant abuses of human rights and political murder.

In 2016, the biggest medical journal in the world, the *Lancet*, did attempt to question Rwanda about this other side to the country's reputation, first with an editorial questioning journalistic freedom in the country and asking whether Rwanda was the complete opposite to the country usually depicted in the journal – a human rights-defending, women's-health success story. In writing his piece, the editor reached out to a Rwandan colleague who allayed his concerns and said that 'surely it would be unreasonable for the cumulative experience of countless medical professionals with deep knowledge of Rwanda gained over many years to be overridden by one mythmaker', the mythmakers here being the sources in the original editorial. Avoiding a clear judgement, the editor concluded the issue needed more scrutiny.[22]

Two years later, the *Lancet* tried again with Pulitzer Prize-winning journalist Laurie Garrett's short 'Perspective' piece reviewing Judi Rever's book *In Praise of Blood: the Crimes of the Rwandan Patriotic Front*, in which Garrett notes, 'Kagame's critics have a funny way of getting into car accidents', and how one physician who worked in the country argues, 'The global health community's love affair with Kagame's Rwanda has to end.'[23] The leader of Rwanda's health transformation, Agnes Binagwaho, wrote a rapid response criticising the article as 'revisionist history' and condemning the *Lancet* for publishing it, as it would not publish a piece on holocaust denial. This may seem like an odd comparison, as the main article never denied the Rwandan genocide, but such an accusation is a core part of Rwanda's authoritarian politics, where anyone seen to criticise the government is accused of genocide denial. What is particularly notable about Binagwaho's rebuttal is the clear example of healthwashing: 'Garrett's Perspective makes no attempt to acknowledge Rwanda's contemporary progress to improve health outcomes.'[24] As if health outcomes absolve the car accidents, as if what everyone should be talking about is the Rwandan success story.

The global health community's love affair with Kagame's Rwanda did not end. More aid, international conferences and high-profile platforms were offered to Rwandan health officials and politicians without so much as a question about the politics of the country. As the world of global health changed after COVID-19, and countries in Africa were demanding greater say on decisions of global health security and vaccine manufacturing, it was Rwanda again that came to the fore in leading these discussions. Once again, the country was using health as a tool of foreign policy, and once again partners could not, and chose not to, ignore Rwanda. Instead, Rwanda expanded its reputation as a country world leaders could do business with. A solution to migration to Europe, a UN 'pacesetter' in solutions to climate change, and a growing presence in international peacekeeping and African security.[25] Through women's health the country had solidified its reputation and future at the heart of global health and African international relations.

Healthwashing and soft power are important places to start thinking about the exploitation of women's health in global politics because they rest on the power of success. Usually when we think about the political exploitation of women's health, we assume it is going to be a negative story, one about governments failing women and their health. Rwanda flips this expectation. Rwanda's approach to women's health and gender equity demonstrates the advances that can be made in women's health when a country sees it as a priority. This is a vital point: governments can transform women's health if they want to. It is not impossible in low-income, post-conflict countries if politicians and health leaders have the right political will, investment and a strategy. Not investing or investing in the wrong type of plan for women's health is rarely based on evidence or financial decisions, but political ones. Transforming women's health is a major win for women and for politicians and can be a major source of soft power in international diplomacy. Promoting women's health is a far more effective tool of foreign policy than curtailing women's health. Given the efficacy of such soft power, it is a wonder more countries don't invest in and exploit women's health in the same way.

2

The Aid Boom and Saving Mothers

Between 2005 and 2006, I spent a lot of time sat in traffic on the road from my local neighbourhood in Kijitonyama to the central business district of Dar es Salaam, Tanzania, staring out of the window of a *dala dala*. On a good day, I would have a squished seat on the bus, but as is the norm with any commute in any major city at rush hour, most of the time I was standing, trying not to think of the sweat down the backs of my legs. My distraction was always what was happening outside the bus. I stared jealously at the white 4x4s of the many UN agencies, as people in the back ruffled through their papers in lovely air conditioning, preparing for meetings about how they were or were not meeting their poverty reduction targets. I tried to keep a mental note of all the large wooden signs we passed for NGOs of various sizes, advertising all the work they were doing to end HIV/AIDS and maternal mortality. No one had smartphones then, so if I wanted to interview someone for my PhD about the governance of HIV/AIDS I'd have to give them a call or remember the turning for where their offices were and try my luck. Everywhere you looked there was a sign, a company building boosting its commitment to healthcare with pictures of mothers holding newborn babies, or a newspaper advert tendering for a new health project sponsored by a European government. Even the *dala dalas* – the local buses like the one I was in, efficiently cutting up the UN's 4x4s – occasionally had positive health messages about maternal health or HIV/AIDS painted on them. It appeared to me that this is what Dar es Salaam was in the business of doing – saving women and children from two of the biggest killers in poor countries like Tanzania: maternal mortality and HIV/AIDS. The aid sector's effort to save mothers was decorating the city. It was a booming industry.

2005 was the beginning of the growth period in foreign aid for health. Not only was the aid money flowing into countries like Tanzania, but some of the biggest aid programmes at the time centred on improving women's health, specifically saving mothers. In 1990, 'development assistance for health', as foreign aid to health is officially categorised, was at an average of US$5.7 billion a year. This had increased to US$13 billion by 2000, but by 2018 it had tripled to a peak of US$39 billion.[1]

Aid donors such as the US and the UK were pouring money into the leading causes of death of young women in poor countries – HIV/AIDS and maternal mortality. Women's health was not an invisible afterthought, forgotten on the sidelines of global politics, it was front and centre as an international priority that all countries got behind. Not only did donors and governments want to fund programmes that targeted women specifically, they also wanted to ensure that it was women in the driving seat.

But these policies ignored many women. If you weren't a mother, had no intention of becoming a mother, a pregnant person or parent, or were a woman unable to reproduce or past reproductive age, you did not figure in this story. Many women's health advocates stress the need to go beyond the bikini issues – women's sexual and reproductive health and breast cancer – but when it came to global financing for women's health in the early 2000s, it didn't even get to the bra. The power of foreign aid did get the international community to focus on women's health, but in doing so it shifted women's health to mean one thing in the world – saving mothers, to the exclusion of all other women and women's other complex health needs.

To understand how foreign aid made women's health all about saving mothers, it is important to begin with thinking around how anti-poverty and development economics shifted from the 1980s to the early 2000s. It was during this period that anti-poverty campaigners began to show how poverty had become increasingly feminised, and foreign aid agencies recognised the potential role poor women could play in delivering major aid programmes.

Throughout the 1980s and early 1990s, women had become the crashmat of the types of macro-economic development policies that dominated anti-poverty thinking in the world. During this period, major international aid agencies and financial institutions such as the World Bank and International Monetary Fund (IMF) were interested in reducing countries' vulnerability to debt and financial crises, and enhancing economic growth by cutting public-sector spending and regulation, and opening up economies to international trade and finance. The idea was that inserting a country into the global economy created new opportunities for growth and investment, and reducing government spending would help balance the books and reduce debt. The more countries aligned to these principles, the more aid money they received from the IMF and World Bank. Restructuring economies around these principles was called structural adjustment or, in the case of post-communist countries in the mid-1990s that saw rapid and blunt applications of these principles, shock therapy. The idea was that economies would be subject to a big shock or high dose of economic medicine, which might hurt in the short term, but would ultimately pay off in the long term once the economy grew. The part that economists did not want you to think about was how people coped with these changes in the short term: most of this 'coping' was done by women acting as economic crashmats to cuts in public spending by taking on extra paid work to make up for shortfalls in household income, and doing additional unpaid labour in family and community care work. At the height of these economic shocks, women in some parts of the world, like East Africa and India, were estimated to be working up to sixteen hours a day. Women were doing two-thirds of the world's work for a tenth of the world's income. As a landmark Commonwealth report on the impacts of structural adjustment on women at the time stated, 'Women are at the epicentre of the crisis and bear the brunt of adjustment efforts.'[2]

Longer term, these economic reforms did not bring about the promised prosperity and growth. Debt increased. As states competed to attract foreign investment, labour standards decreased. This had a direct impact on women in the labour market because they were seen as cheaper and easier to exploit, as at the time they were perceived as less likely to be members of unions and more likely to have dependants needing their wage. A growth in the import of foreign goods saw increases in food imports, which often out-priced domestic farmers and food producers. This again affected women who worked in informal agricultural labour in poor countries and vendors of local produce who struggled to compete with foreign imports. Health services were opened up to foreign competition and investment, and in turn saw cuts in public-sector investment in health and welfare provision. This increased out-of-pocket expenditure for individuals accessing healthcare, and weakened health systems in poor countries as they did not have the funds to sustain them. Public services and welfare went into decline. The private sector did not fill the void, especially not in health and social care. Women did.

Cuts to public-sector spending and welfare (economic austerity) create gaps in social care provisioning that are filled by women in the home and wider community. The way this works starts at the end of a twelve-hour shift in low-paid manufacturing or agricultural work. You walk home or maybe take the bus if you have extra cash that week. As soon as you get home, you feed your children and make sure they have attended school that day, before sitting down with the elderly relatives who live with you to check they have taken their medicine and have also eaten. You then leave the house to run errands for your family, attend a community meeting or go door to door collecting and distributing food for those in need, or checking in with neighbours undergoing a bout of ill health – be it from malaria, cholera or HIV – perhaps topping up their water, changing their bedsheets and taking the dirty washing home with you to clean and return. When you get home you clean up, check your daughter will be able to get the rest of your children ready for school the next day – that's if your children are of school age; if not, your eldest daughter will stay off school to look after them while you go to work. This is an economic calculation: you know your son will be likely to get a higher-paid job than your daughter, so better to keep him in school if there is a choice. If there is food left over, you sit down and eat before going to bed. This is what is called the triple burden faced by women: the first burden is the paid work, the second burden is the family and household and the third burden is picking up the social and healthcare gaps left by economic austerity. This triple burden is intergenerational: from a young age, daughters know to pick up the slack, learning that it is their responsibility to do so. If this sounds similar to the type of impact austerity measures had in high-income countries after the 2008 financial crisis, then it is: same patterns, just different extremes, depending on the wealth and welfare of the country in which these mechanisms are imposed and the scale of economic cuts.

To top all of this, women are often the direct beneficiaries of welfare support, such as child benefits, and the jobs created by public provisioning, such as paid work in the health and care sector. These cuts therefore affect women's household income and work. As a final insult, economic restructuring was presented as an opportunity for women, one in which they could gain economic autonomy through greater employment opportunities outside the home. However, these opportunities came at a wider cost to their health and well-being from respiratory diseases caused by the noxious fumes inhaled in factories, to intense limb pain arising from long working hours, and controlled and limited use of the loo.

By the end of the 1990s, more and more countries were complaining to the World Bank and IMF that this approach was not working for them. They were in debt. Cuts to public-sector budgets were having negative impacts on health and education. And the elusive growth was either not happening, and/or definitely not trickling down to the whole of the country. Women were exhausting themselves from picking up the slack where public provisions were absent and gender inequality, particularly economic inequality, persisted. These governments were looking elsewhere for loans and assistance. This alarmed those working in the World Bank and the IMF. If no one wanted to borrow from them, they would no longer have a job. And if the major states that paid into these institutions and kept them going weren't seeing results, they would stop funding them. Activists wanted change. Countries wanted change. Even people who worked for the World Bank and IMF wanted change. Feminists around the world joined campaigns against development agencies and their structural adjustment policies, arguing that they'd had more than enough of women being the face of the most extreme forms of poverty, being asked to do more and more with less and less. Development experts began arguing for a shift away from big economic restructuring projects as a means to end poverty, to more 'human development' projects that prioritised specific issues – health, education, sanitation, gender equality – which would target the needs of the poor. At the core of these needs were the basics: stop newborn babies from dying, stop malnutrition and, crucially, improve the health of women to keep mothers alive. Things had to change.

Enter the Millennium Development Goals (MDGs). In September 2000, all member states signed up to the UN Millennium Declaration, a commitment to peace, security and disarmament, protecting the environment, human rights, strengthening the UN and noting the 'special needs' of Africa. One aspect of the declaration, 'Development and Poverty Eradication', outlined a set of commitments to halve poverty by 2015 that would move away from the macro restructuring of economies of the 1980s and early 1990s, to prioritising the issues that kept people in poverty – ill health, lack of education, gender inequality – and do something about them. The idea was that if you could compile a list of all the main scourges in the world, get governments to agree on a set of goals and progress indicators, you could give a focus to foreign aid spending and enact real change in ending poverty. This list ultimately became the eight MDGs. Of the eight MDGs, one goal focused on gender equality and women's empowerment (Goal 3), one goal *explicitly* targeted women's health by committing the world to improving maternal health (Goal 5) and one goal directly addressed the leading cause of death of young women in the world, HIV/AIDS (Goal 6). The goals were a clear recognition of the disproportionate impact of poverty on women and girls and, more than that, an acknowledgment that it is the health of women and girls that directly contributes to their poverty. Like Rwanda in the last chapter, the international community knew that to fix poverty, you needed to prioritise the health of women and girls.

All UN commitments involve a great deal of compromise. The compromise for women's health in the new MDG era was that the focus would be on maternal health, not sexual and reproductive health. In other words, they took out the part of women's health the majority of governments in the world seek to restrict: abortion and contraception. Women's health advocates would get their goal – Goal 5 to improve maternal mortality – but without commitment to address some of the major causes of maternal mortality, notably lack of access to safe abortion and modern contraception, they would be trying to end maternal mortality with their dominant hand tied behind their back. Some in the donor community were talking about this, but most were reticent to push it, not wanting to upset the likes of Saudi Arabia, Vatican City and the US. Women's health advocates, policy specialists and clinicians had entered a Faustian pact with aid donors: they could get the money for *some* aspects of women's health – ending maternal mortality – but doing so diverted money and political attention away from some of the other major killers of women – most obviously lack of access to abortion, but also other big killers such as heart and respiratory diseases. When you work for decades on an issue that is continuously overlooked and under-funded and you see thousands of women die from preventable causes, you can see why a compromise to get some action is better than nothing. But these compromises and priorities were not due to politicians, policy-makers and aid agencies not knowing that all the evidence pointed to comprehensive sex education, modern contraception and safe abortion as the best way of protecting women and girls from preventable death from pregnancy, childbirth or AIDS. They knew. But the focus of the MDGs was never about overall women's health: it was always about saving mothers.

The reason for this is simple: saving mothers appeals to governments in the UN, voters, aid givers and society at large because saving mothers equals saving babies. Governments, the UN, charities and most people in the world are united around giving babies and young children the best chance in life. One of the best ways of ensuring newborn babies survive to the age of five (the cut-off point for what counts as child mortality) is making sure their mothers survive. For aid-giving politicians, saving mothers and babies is a good way of justifying your aid budget to tax payers, because saving mothers and babies has greater appeal to the voting public than other forms of aid spending. Building a road, for example (which is actually quite helpful for mothers, who benefit like the rest of the population from effective infrastructure spending), is harder to sell to the tax payer than saving mothers and babies. For aid recipients, saving mothers is a key way of signalling your investment in the future of the country, women's health and gender equality, and your commitment to family life and values.

But 'save mothers, save babies' is only part of the story. The other compelling reason to save mothers is they will work hard for you. They will raise the kids, go to work and invest in your country's future. As global philanthropist Melinda French Gates put it, if you invest in women, they will invest in everyone else.[3] Governments and aid agencies know that saving mothers is not just about what you can do for them, but also about what they can do for you. Give mothers the opportunity and investment and they can raise a family and a whole country out of poverty. You may have thought like this yourself, looking at the mums around you multi-tasking and thinking if they were just given some sleep and power they could work out all the world's problems. By the early 2000s, policy-makers and anti-poverty thinkers were thinking just like you, and started putting their money where the mothers were. The invest-in-mothers mantra had gone from political rhetoric to a 'quiet revolution'[4] in ending poverty and improving health outcomes in the global south.

The quiet revolution referred to new social welfare and protection schemes that concentrated on transferring money directly to the pockets of the poor. Some of the schemes were similar to traditional child benefit models of regular payments to mothers based on the age and number of children they have. These are much like the child allowance my mum got in England in the 1980s, when proof of my existence was enough to receive the cash. The difference with modern cash transfers is most are conditional on mothers proving that their children are putting on weight, going to school regularly or attending clinics for health checks and vaccinations. Two of the most famous cash-transfer schemes in the world launched in the early 2000s – Progresa-Oportunidades in Mexico and Bolsa Família in Brazil – specifically targeted mothers and female heads of the household as the main recipients of the cash. The overriding sense of all of this was that if you just give women money they will know what to do with it and help the international community reach their development targets. Women could be trusted to engage with the programme and spend the additional welfare funds on their children. Men, in contrast, rarely came off well in such policy planning: fathers were seen to be absent, unreliable or untrustworthy, and risked spending the welfare payments on themselves, whereas evidence showed that when women had money they would spend it on their children.

There is a lot to unpack about the gender stereotypes and problems around such assumptions. Not all men are terrible fathers. Leaving fathers out of the equation reinforces the idea that they don't have to look after or be responsible for their kids, and that childcare and child health is solely women's work. Numerous academic studies have been conducted on the impact of cash transfers on shifting power relations within the family. Is it good for women? Does it put women at more or less risk of intimate-partner violence? The results are mixed. As many leading development experts such as the late Sylvia Chant have decried, the whole thing smacks of women *yet again* taking on an additional burden: not only are they subject to extreme poverty, now they are responsible for ending it. But, of course, given the opportunity, when it came to spending the cash transfers wisely, they did.

All the evidence is cash transfers work. Women do spend the cash on their families. Cash transfers lead to significant improvement in nutrition and school attendance, break cycles of intergenerational poverty and stimulate economic growth as the poor have money to spend in the economy. Bolsa Família has been credited with a reduction from 28 per cent of Brazilians living in poverty, a fixed number for most of the 1990s, to 17 per cent in 2008, with child malnutrition in the poorest region of the country falling by 45 per cent.[5]

Politicians such as Brazil's charismatic on (2003–2011) and off (to jail 2018–19) and on again (2023–) President Luiz Inácio 'Lula' da Silva were only too happy to own the success of what mothers and female heads of households had achieved, and share with aid agencies and other countries what they could learn from countries like Brazil. Aid agencies and governments went mad for it. In the 2000s, for many working in the global south, cash transfers to mothers were the revolution that was going to change development programmes and end poverty for ever. They cropped up throughout the world from welfare programmes that began in the late 1990s in South Africa, China and Indonesia, to child benefit initiatives in Peru, Jamaica and Mongolia, to the standard cash transfers for school and health clinic attendance in the Philippines, Bangladesh and Cambodia. In 2006, the African Union declared cash-transfer programmes so effective that every African country should have one. The World Bank even trialled a cash-transfer programme where they paid young women in Tanzania and Malawi to stay HIV negative, the idea being the cash would replace the incentive for young women to have sex with sugar daddies. Give mothers the money and watch poverty end. Women, and mothers in particular, would be the engines of development: the key to the success of anti-poverty and child health programmes. To drive countries out of poverty, you needed healthy mothers.

A focus on giving money to mothers is one thing, but prioritising women's health means very little unless governments and aid donors are willing to stump up the cash needed to do it properly. The first fifteen years of the new millennium were marked by unprecedented funding for women's health issues in foreign aid. Foreign aid for health issues predominantly came from three sources during this time – the US government, the UK government and the Bill & Melinda Gates Foundation. According to OECD (Organisation for Economic Co-operation and Development) data (the main source for monitoring the billions of dollars that go into aid spending and how much is spent), spending on the category that covers sexual and reproductive health including HIV/ AIDS, 'Population policies, programmes, and reproductive health' doubled between 2005 and 2015, from a total of US$6.1 billion to US$12.2 billion per year, with US$152.6 billion spent over ten years.

The vast majority of funds – US$111.1 billion – was spent on HIV/AIDS programming.[6] The majority of people living with HIV/AIDS in the world are women, AIDS is the leading cause of death of young women in the world, and one woman is infected with HIV every minute. HIV/AIDS was where the blockbuster health projects were at, and women – or, you guessed it, specifically mothers – were a central part of those projects.

The biggest of all the programmes during this time was US President George W. Bush's President's Emergency Plan for AIDS Relief (PEPFAR). PEPFAR is a $100 billion project. It is the largest amount of funding given to HIV/AIDS, or any single health issue for that matter, from any country in the world. Set up in 2003, it is one presidential initiative that has consistently seen the support of both Democrat and Republican presidents. Even Donald Trump kept up support for PEPFAR.

In 2003, 40 million people were estimated to live with HIV, 5 million had contracted the virus and 3 million people had died from AIDS in that one year. Of these numbers, 700,000 new infections and 500,000 deaths were children.[7] Bush wanted to save pregnant women and innocent children from HIV. Women and pregnant people can prevent the transmission of HIV to their baby by taking the drug Nevirapine when pregnant and following breastfeeding guidelines. The problem in the early 2000s was that Nevirapine was not widely available to pregnant people living with HIV, and neither was access to the breastfeeding guidelines or breast milk substitutes. This is a problem the Bush government thought it could solve.

For Bush, there was the good HIV-positive person – the innocent child or pregnant woman; and then there were the bad HIV-positive people – drug users and sex workers. He did not want US aid dollars going to support the purchase, distribution and promotion of condoms or interventions that targeted vulnerable groups such as intravenous drug users. The battle against HIV/AIDS would be won by promoting family values, abstinence, monogamy and providing a massive scale up for access to treatment. The programme would focus on the AB – Abstain, Be faithful (no 'C' for condoms) – of prevention and access to treatment using drugs procured from US pharmaceutical companies. People living with HIV get drugs for free, US government subsidises US industry, pharmaceutical companies make a profit.

Being able to stop mothers passing on HIV to their babies was seen as a major win by the US government and the wider donor community: it stopped babies being born with HIV and helped improve the health of mothers as they would be tested and put on antiretroviral treatment, and keeping mothers healthy was vital for healthy babies. Keeping mothers and babies alive was something that could be easily measured and aligned with the priorities and preferences of the governments that were pumping money into foreign aid. An added bonus was that it did great work for the reputation of politicians such as Bush and the US government. Sure, he made colossal mistakes with the War on Terror, but just look at what he did for mothers living with HIV/AIDS around the world.

PEPFAR changed the game of getting people living with HIV onto treatment. Like it or loathe it, it was the first programme that got people in need on to treatment and helped them live. When I first started to research the HIV/AIDS crisis in 2004, people were dying, at home, with the support of just their friends, family and local community, and without any treatment. Pregnant women were unable to access treatment to prevent the transmission of HIV to their babies. Babies were being born with HIV when they didn't have to be. While there was considerable activism around this, notably from the incredible South African-based Treatment Action Campaign (TAC), it was the influx of PEPFAR money that created immediate change. PEPFAR did three really noticeable things. First, it stopped people dying. People could live with HIV. Second, it showed that it was possible to run a major treatment campaign for people living with HIV in poor settings. I have lost count of the number of times someone has told me you can't do something in poor communities because of a lack of infrastructure, education and – according to the ex-head of USAID Andrew Natsios – the inability of Africans to tell the time (this casual racism is not consigned to the past: similar arguments were made about COVID-19 vaccines in Africa). Third, it created a clustering effect of aid towards women, specifically mothers living with HIV.

While PEPFAR was undoubtedly the biggest bilateral health programme in the world, it was accompanied by multiple other million-dollar programmes from other aid agencies targeting women. The more money that leading donors such as the US put into saving mothers, preventing the transmission of HIV from mother to baby and prioritising prevention in young women, the more other donors – both public and private – got on board. The amount of money going towards HIV/ AIDS during the early 2000s was such that the international community set up an independent funding mechanism – the Global Fund to Fight AIDS, Tuberculosis and Malaria – to help sustain and channel all of this money to the countries and communities that needed it.

Investing in two or three aspects of health leaves governments to fill the gap of everything else. People tend to think that most health financing in poor countries comes from donors: not true. Aid does help, but the majority of health financing in many poor countries comes from their own governments. And like donor clustering, government funding tends to map on to trends in aid funding. This is because donors want to see governments step up and match their funding, or take 'ownership' of a specific health project. It is also because these governments are on the hook for meeting the targets set by the international community in the MDGs. As the Rwanda model showed, political commitment and ownership of national health programmes and key targets were central to driving change. Low- and middle-income countries like Tanzania,

where we began this chapter, receive more aid depending on
how they can show results on key targets – for example, the
number of women who gave birth in a clinic. The more they
hit the target, the more aid money flows in. Hence, the more
you invest your own government funds towards an issue, the
more likely you are to hit the target and get the top-up cash.
Like Rwanda, you are now best in class: aid money rewards
progress, saving mothers suggests your country is developing,
development attracts foreign investment, foreign investment
helps you get rich, everyone's a winner. Ish. Women who want
to have children and people living with HIV/AIDS win out;
everyone else not so much.

At the height of the spending to save mothers in 2012, if you
lived in a small rural community in a country like Tanzania,
the HIV/AIDS treatment centre and maternal and newborn
health clinic were often side by side and probably the only
official health centres in your region. These clinics were built
with the aid money that flowed towards the MDGs from
major programmes like PEPFAR in the early 2000s. I am a
big fan of these clinics, officially because they became a vital
resource for people living with HIV during a terrible period
in the AIDS crisis, but really because I am a sucker for seeing
babies being weighed in slings. For some rural communities,
these next-door HIV and baby clinics were the nearest health
facility for hundreds of miles. If you were HIV positive and/or
pregnant or a new mum, your health needs were met by health
experts at these clinics. But for every other health issue: nothing. If you were sick for any other reason, you would visit the
duka la dawa – the pharmacist – to buy antibiotics, or borrow
money to travel to the nearest big town with a hospital.

Far from being a limit on your life, having an HIV status
could open up a range of provisions that would otherwise
be unavailable to you, from nutritional programmes to peer

educational activities to seed funding for business ideas. This distorts how you think about your health and even pregnancy. As one person suggested to me, maybe they should contract HIV, or at the very least pretend to, as a means to access these resources. It also distorts how health is delivered in a rural community. Everything shifts to where the money is. If you were an enterprising health official or politician, you would use aid money to build a clinic in your town. You might also use some of the funds earmarked for HIV/AIDS or maternal health to fund other aspects of health in the area. This would be a creative use of a budget line. If you showed good progress and indicators on maternal deaths in the area, this would lead to an increase in funding. Saving mothers through HIV/AIDS and maternal health projects thus became an income stream to support local health initiatives. If a town, region or country could prove it was dealing with maternal mortality and HIV well, then more money and investment would come. Saving mothers was a means of attracting and sustaining donor aid money. As all the NGO signs and 4x4s of the Dar es Salaam morning commute showed at the start of this chapter, it was big business.

This skewing of a health sector towards saving mothers is an example of what public health specialists call the vertical/horizontal debate. Donors want to fund specific 'vertical' issues, like saving mothers, but don't want to fund 'horizontal' issues that cut across all healthcare, notably health systems that cater to a range of health issues women may face. This is a major problem for any aid-reliant country. Imagine building a health system around two priority issues, say breast cancer and heart disease – good for some women, but leaves a lot else under-funded. Throw into the mix the fact that these issues are not defined by you, or the politicians you elect, but by experts from outside your country, and you can see the problem. For women's health, it means a huge distortion towards saving mothers, and pretty much nothing on the other major killers of women in the world, namely so-called non-communicable diseases (NCDs) such as heart disease, stroke, dementia, diabetes, cancer, respiratory infections and lung disease, and one of the leading causes of death and bad health in poor countries: diarrhoeal diseases. There is so little data on health spending in these areas that the OECD only started publishing it in 2018, by which point US$25 million in aid money had been spent *in total* in one year on NCDs – so that includes all cancers, tobacco-related NCDs, heart disease and mental health – which grew to US$163 million in 2019 once donors started to recognise this was a problem.[8] To reiterate, that is US$163 million in aid spending to cover all of those major causes of death of women throughout all aid-recipient countries. Contrast that with the US$4.7 *billion* spent on HIV/AIDS in the same year and you start to get my point: funding was going to some women's health issues, but completely neglecting others.

By the 2015 deadline of the MDGs, the warnings around maternal mortality and HIV/AIDS had been heeded. In 2000, globally 451,000 women and girls died of pregnancy and birth-related complications.[9] In 2015, it was 303,000 women and girls. If the aim was to save mothers, a 34.4 per cent decline in maternal mortality most definitely showed progress. Maternal mortality had received attention and money, and was slowly in decline. Women also no longer had to worry about passing HIV on to their children. Prevention of mother to child transmission of HIV is one of the biggest success stories in global health, seeing a 70 per cent reduction between 2000 and 2015. In 2000, an estimated 490,000 children were born with HIV; by 2015 this had reduced to 150,000.[10] The international community showed it could act on women's health if it chose to.

After the height of spending in 2018, development assistance for health started to decrease as aid donors shifted priorities, new leaders came to power and rich countries faced their own austerity cuts. One of the biggest funding reductions was on maternal mortality. Even funding for HIV/AIDS – an area of health spending that many thought would be protected in development budgets – was starting to wane. In 2015, the MDGs were replaced by seventeen Sustainable Development Goals (SDGs) that kept a goal focused on gender equality, but lumped all health issues into one 'health and well-being' goal. The health and well-being goal kept the same HIV/AIDS, maternal mortality and child mortality targets as the MDGs, and added reproductive health – although this was still sufficiently vague for countries to interpret or limit as they saw fit. Technically, these issues were still a priority for the international community, but they were competing with even more priorities, claims to resources and a new decade of high-level global crises and economic instability. With the shift from the old to the new goals, all aspects of foreign aid to health, with the exception of health emergencies, started to dip.

By 2021, 295,650 women around the world were still dying every year from pregnancy- and birth-related complications. That's 810 women a day, or one woman every two minutes. This number has been stagnant since 2016. Governments and international agencies still said in 2023 that getting this number down further was a major political priority, but such commitments were rarely backed up with the necessary finances or comprehensive strategies. After decades of a focus on human development and women's health, economists and politicians around the world once more started to obsess over growth and macro restructuring of economies.

The 2000s marked a critical turning point in women's health around the world. Saving mothers had become a global political priority, as had getting mothers to save everyone else. Invest in them and their health, give them money to make sure their kids eat well and go to school, and the world will transform. But, of course, women's health only mattered with reference to motherhood and what women could do for everyone else. Unless women were mothers or HIV positive, the world did not care about their health. This set a dangerous precedent whereby any future investment in women's health has to be justified by claims of return – for example, invest in breast cancer screenings and keep women alive during their prime earning potential, address heart disease in women so they can live longer and help look after the grandkids, invest in women and they will become better doctors and cure every cancer ... Look around you: these sorts of justifications are everywhere. When we say women's health matters for any other reason than women themselves, we devalue the lives and health of women. As the next chapter will show, time and again politicians use the idea that women only have value as mothers to win votes and restrict women's health, with deadly consequences for women.

3

Hard Power and the Global Gag Rule

On 23 January 2017, one week after his inauguration, Donald Trump sat down at the large, polished desk in the Oval Office of the White House. Over his left shoulder stood eight white men in suits, and over his right shoulder, another white man in a suit, his vice president, Mike Pence. One woman was tacked on to the side of this gathering, as if someone at the last minute thought adding a woman would be a good idea. Most of the white men in suits wore the smirk-smile of people excited to be beside a new president at work. One of the men, the White House chief strategist, Steve Bannon, wore the biggest smile as he watched Trump open the leather folder in front of him, pick up his pen and, with a serious look in his eye, sign the executive order into law. After signing the single-page document, Trump turned the opened folder, pen still in hand, to show the assembled press. As one of the first acts of his presidency, he had signed the Mexico City Policy – aka the global gag rule – back into law. This one act would have devastating consequences for the health and lives of women around the world.

The global gag rule is the most glaring example of the US imposing its ideology on other countries while simultaneously undermining international commitments to stopping women from dying when they don't have to. Named after the city where the 1984 United Nations Conference on Population and Development took place, the Mexico City Policy is a flagship foreign policy of the Republican party. The rule is clear: no organisation abroad in receipt of US funds for family planning and reproductive health can conduct abortions or talk about them, hence its 'global gag rule' moniker. The impact is huge: millions of dollars of aid to sexual and reproductive health cut, projects cancelled overnight, longstanding partnerships ruined and vulnerable women at risk of death at the whim of a decision made by a US Republican president thousands of miles away.

Abortion has long been a tool of global hard power with deadly consequences for women, and the US is one of the best countries in showing how this works. In contrast to soft power explored in Chapter 1, hard power refers to explicit ways in which one country or power may coerce or change what is happening in another. Coercion in global politics can be achieved through military interventions, economic sanctions, diplomatic bargaining and, in this case, economic sanctions on women's health. Here, the US government is not using its classic hard power resources – its vast military, trade deals or intelligence networks – to bend the world to its interests, but women's health.

Since the Mexico City Policy was passed in 1984 by Ronald Reagan, every Democrat president has reversed the global gag rule as one of his first acts, and every Republican president has reinstated it. This back and forth is less to do with changing attitudes to women's health around the world than with domestic US politics. The global gag rule builds on two prior acts of US federal legislation: the 1973 Helms Amendment, which blocks US aid from funding abortion as a form of family planning, and the 1981 Siljander Amendment, which bans foreign aid going towards lobbying for or against abortion. Both of these were enacted in reaction to Roe vs Wade in 1973, a Supreme Court ruling that protected American women's right to abortion under the constitution until it was overturned in 2022. The less politicians were able to restrict abortion within America itself, the more they looked to restrict women's access to abortion around the world. In doing so, politicians could appeal to those in the American electorate who were against abortion by showing they were taking a stand globally, thus building international and domestic support for the ultimate political long game of overturning Roe.

Republican presidents don't just reinstate the global gag rule when they come to power; to really prove their chops, they extend it. Curtailing women's health is used as bragging rights. In 2017, Trump extended the coverage of the gag, re-naming it the not so catchy but even more deadly 'Protecting Life in Global Health Assistance' (PLGHA) rule, so the gag applied to any organisation in receipt of aid money for global health, including UN agencies. This meant that it was not just NGOs receiving US funds that would be gagged: in effect, Trump was gagging the UN. If the UN health organisations wanted to receive US money they would have to cease funding or talking about abortion. That is, the entirety of the UN in the entirety of the world.

Trump did not stop there. To make sure he was truly scuppering the UN's efforts to prevent women from dying in pregnancy and childbirth, and to give them choice over their reproductive lives, he cut all funds to the UN's main sexual and reproductive health organisation: the UN Population Fund (UNFPA). He was able to do this under the 1985 Kemp-Kasten Amendment, which stops funds going to any organisation *that the president determines* is supporting involuntary sterilisation or coercive abortion. Even if there is no evidence that an organisation is doing either of these things – and evaluations by the US government have found no evidence of this – if the president thinks it is, then it doesn't get the cash. To get a sense of the scale of the global gag rule under Trump, under George W. Bush the global gag *only* (and I use the term lightly) applied to the $600 million the US government spent every year on sexual and reproductive health. Under Trump, the extension meant it applied to the $9 billion the US government spent on global health programmes every year.

Under Trump's extended gag, MSI Reproductive Choices, one of the biggest women's health organisations in the world, saw a 17 per cent, or $30 million, reduction in aid. According to the charity, 'Continued USAID funding would have allowed MSI to serve an estimated 8 million women with family planning, preventing an estimated 6 million unintended pregnancies, 1.8 million unsafe abortions, and 20,000 maternal deaths.'[1]

When Trump announced the extension, other countries stepped up their contribution to sexual and reproductive health aid to try and fill the billion-dollar gap. Canada, Sweden, Finland and the Bill & Melinda Gates Foundation pledged an additional $21 million, and the Netherlands, Luxembourg and Belgium an additional $11 million. The UK, one of the biggest donors to women's health, maintained its $250 million budget commitment.[2] But, of course, these additional pledges could do very little to compete with the average annual funding of $600 million on sexual and reproductive health from the US government, let alone the $9 billion to global health programmes. It was not enough to offset the disaster for women's health. As Vanessa Rios of the International Women's Health Coalition put it, 'Girls are dying because of this rule.'[3]

*

Unsafe abortion and lack of pregnancy loss care is one of the leading causes of maternal mortality in the world. Abortion bans don't stop abortions. They just increase the risk and cost of abortion. Take, for example, a Guttmacher Institute study on the impact of George W. Bush's resurrection of the gag rule in Ghana. In this period of the global gag rule, rural Ghana saw a 12 per cent increase in pregnancies, with between 300,000 and 750,000 unplanned births, and an *additional* (i.e. in contrast to the number of abortions in the years outside of this period) 200,000 abortions.[4] According to a 2019 study published in the *Lancet Global Health*, far from stopping abortion, rates of abortion in African countries affected by the global gag rule under George W. Bush *increased*.[5] If you want to reduce the number of unwanted pregnancies and abortions in the world, abortion bans are not the way to go about it. The effective way of doing it is through free safe and modern contraception, education and economic progress for women, comprehensive sex education, and promoting gender equality in domestic laws and policies. However, bans on these measures – notably comprehensive sex education and access to safe and modern contraception – often accompany abortion bans and are indirectly affected by the global gag rule.

The organisations that run abortion and information services targeted by the global gag rule tend to cover all aspects of sexual and reproductive health, including contraception advice and provision, community outreach work and HIV/AIDS services. Many are specialists in sexual and reproductive health for LGBTQ+ people. Health provision for such marginalised and stigmatised (and, in some instances, criminalised) people and communities can take years of trust and relationship building. Gagging these organisations not only impacts on abortion and wider sexual and reproductive health, but also leads to cuts in vital services and breakdowns in long-term community partnerships that serve the health needs of some of the most marginalised people in the world.

It is not only the marginalised minority who are affected. The global gag rule has led to the closure of core, everyday health facilities and community outreach programmes, cuts to services depending on what can and can't be funded under the strict criteria, and governments and doctors being in constant fear of upsetting the US president and having their funding cut. One health official in Zimbabwe put the problem in stark terms: he had to make a choice between sustenance and values. Do you accept support from the US and abandon your values and commitments to women in your country, or do you starve your policies and programmes but stick to what you know is the right thing to do, and scrabble to get by somehow? It is an impossible question. Pregnancy and birth complications are the leading cause of death for girls and women aged between fifteen and forty-nine in Zimbabwe.[6] You can't bring down maternal mortality without providing access to contraception and safe abortion. Which means you can't address the leading cause of death for women in Zimbabwe when you are being gagged on the very same things that stop them from dying. But you also need funds from the international donors that support the rest of the country's health system and wider anti-poverty programmes. Maternal mortality was a serious issue in an aid-dependent country like Zimbabwe before the gag, but after the Trump gag, health officials were in an impossible position.

All this disruption, chaos and death for a foreign policy that could never achieve its aim in practice: as long as people can get pregnant, people will need abortions.

In an attempt to reduce the death and destruction of the global gag rule, reproductive justice activists monitor the behaviour of the US and recipient governments in implementing the policy. Reproductive justice activists know every letter of the law when it comes to the global gag rule and any other form of abortion legislation, be it domestic or global, and try to stop the over-implementation of the gag rule.

The gag has two prominent exemptions: life endangerment and rape. Talking about abortion under the gag is not illegal, it is restricted – an important, life-saving difference. Such exceptions give space for pushback and defend safe abortion services. The job of activists is to ensure governments, doctors and medical professionals offering abortion are aware of such exemptions and, crucially, are not punished by the law for doing their job. For example, while a doctor may be aware that abortion is permitted for a patient due to a risk to their life, as recognised in domestic law and the global gag rule, they may be unwilling to carry out the procedure or supply pills because of a concern they will be arrested and imprisoned. In countries with laws restricting abortion, third parties assisting a woman to get an abortion face punishment that is often more punitive than those imposed on the person seeking the abortion. In Malawi, for example, a woman who brings about 'miscarriage' (as abortion is labelled in the country's penal code – you can see from this label alone what women in the country are dealing with) can face up to seven years in prison, while someone assisting with a surgical abortion can face fourteen years.[7]

In most countries in which abortion is banned, post-abortion care is not illegal. This may seem confusing but post-abortion care is a whole politics in itself. In countries where abortion is restricted, many women don't want to seek out post-abortion care in case they are reported for abortion, irrespective of whether they had an induced abortion or spontaneously miscarried. Those who do seek post-abortion care after having an abortion may simply state they have miscarried. But such claims in turn mean that sometimes women who spontaneously miscarry are accused of having had illegal abortions, and in extreme cases – such as the over 180 women in prison in El Salvador – face severe punishment. Hence even post-abortion care rules, that help women access the care that they badly need, can create high-stakes threats to their freedom and well-being. Domestic abortion laws and the global gag rule combine to have a chilling effect on the lives of women, governments and the medical profession.

Legal sexual and reproductive rights activists such as the Center for Reproductive Rights work hard to stop this abuse of the law. They hold governments and medical professionals to account and educate them about the limits and exemptions to the law. They also provide legal support where women seeking abortion and those assisting them have been arrested and/ or prosecuted, and pursue high-profile cases where authorities have acted outside the law to prosecute those seeking abortion and those who assist them. The purpose of these cases is not only to seek justice for those affected by incorrect or over-application of the law, but to push for constitutional reform in countries where restrictions on abortion persist. Using the law can be highly effective, but it does not always change the attitudes of (predominantly) men in power.

Given the chilling chaos, disruption and deadly consequences of the global gag rule, one obvious question is why do governments go along with it? Why do they allow this foreign rule to cause so much damage in their countries? Surely it would be better just to decline the US aid and work with other donors to develop programmes? US aid money and good diplomatic reasons are undoubtedly a major part of this. But the real reason is the majority of countries in the world have some type of restriction or limit on abortion. The global gag rule is an effective tool of foreign policy because it connects with the electoral strategies of other men in suits in presidential offices, or seeking presidential office, around the world.

*

According to the Center for Reproductive Rights, 60 per cent of women and pregnant people in the world have access to 'broadly legal' abortion, abortion available on social or economic grounds, loosely based on their income, support networks and living environment, in addition to physical or mental health, subject to gestational limits (the norm being twelve weeks).[8] To look at it from a seriously glass-half-empty point of view, this means nearly half the women in the world have no, or very restricted, access to abortion. As of 2023, seventy-two countries have 'broadly legal' access to abortion, fifty countries permit abortion only when the health of the woman is at risk and twenty-four countries ban abortion completely. Maddeningly, 111 million, or 6 per cent of, women in the world live in countries with total abortion bans.[9] I apologise for repeating myself and shouting, but it is necessary at this point: ABORTION BANS DO NOT STOP ABORTIONS. Instead, they increase the risk of women dying. Politicians know this, yet persist. Why?

A common response to this question is religion. During the 1990s, every time activists and experts pushed to protect the right to abortion in the UN, it was blocked by right-wing religious groups. Religion – specifically the power of the Vatican and the Catholic Church, and Islamic organisations such as the Muslim World League and Muslim World Congress – directly contributed to what is known as the Cairo Compromise within the UN. The 1994 International Conference on Population and Development in Cairo was the first time women's sexual and reproductive rights were officially recognised as a global priority to be protected and upheld by member states of the UN. While Cairo was a major milestone in women's health, and the progress it made should undoubtedly be seen as significant, it rested on a major compromise: advocates of sexual and reproductive rights had to acquiesce to right-wing religious groups and leave out explicit mention of abortion. As we saw with the MDGs in the last chapter, this set a precedent within the UN that still shapes how states commit to women's health, with a narrow focus on saving mothers without mention of abortion. It also set an important precedent within the women's movement, specifically among Black feminists, who led the pushback on how such compromises were narrowing women's reproductive freedom. Finally, in keeping with the theme of exceptionalism around women's health in politics, blocking abortion in the Cairo Declaration in 1994 was an example of Islamic organisations and the Catholic Church agreeing on something and working together in global politics.

Religion is certainly behind some of the most stringent abortion bans in individual countries around the world, such as El Salvador, where, as I noted earlier, abortion is completely banned, and at best carries an eight-year prison term for women seeking or suspected to have had an abortion and, at worst, thirty to fifty years in prison where such women are accused of 'aggravated homicide'. Catholicism is also behind moves to reverse progress on abortion, despite popular support to the contrary, in countries such as Poland. The only Muslim country with an outright ban on abortion is Iraq, but Indonesia, Afghanistan, Iran and Syria all have tightly controlled laws that permit abortion *only* to save a person's life. However, changes to abortion legislation in Argentina in 2020 and Ireland in 2018 show clear signs of progress the other way: that Catholic countries can respond to the will of the people and provide and protect access to safe abortion.

The second answer is, it's the economy, stupid. At times of economic uncertainty, politicians look to mobilise their base around something other than jobs and wealth, appealing to nostalgia and a bygone age and shifting the blame to others for the state of the economy. Politicians blame others for the fact you don't have a job or can't afford to repay your mortgage, be it migrants taking your job, affirmative action schemes that promote under-represented people, or the woke liberals living in cities who want to stop you eating beef burgers and are undermining the economy by rejecting traditional farming. Blaming the other is the first line of populist politics, followed by asserting the idea that (usually wealthy) politicians know what real people want and need. The second line is to prove you're a person of the people by appealing to nostalgia and tradition based on an imaginary past, when life was simple and everyone knew and understood conservative values: the nuclear heterosexual family, the male breadwinner and faith. Outlawing abortion is at the centre of these values. If someone cannot provide for a child, other (predominantly but not limited to) Christian families can adopt and provide that child with love. There is no reason to have an abortion when you put the family at the centre of society, and that society pledges to help you care for the child. The family, not abortion, is the solution. These values are not new to economic crises; religious groups have held some of these beliefs throughout history – the only difference is when politicians connect these beliefs to trends in wider society; for example, during periods of social change when people tether certainty or identity to traditional ideas around the family, family values and gender roles of men and women in the family. The politics comes in when politicians and political movements construe such identities as being under threat, a way of life that is to be defended, and that thing attacking you and your way of life is abortion, and its common ally, LGBTQ+ rights.

Such beliefs appeal to voters during periods of uncertainty, turbulence and economic downturns. Combine this with faith and the billions of dollars right-wing groups put into spreading misinformation about abortions – that abortion is never necessary to save a mother's life (I repeat for the third time, unsafe abortion is a leading cause of maternal mortality), that late-term abortion is common (not true: only 1 per cent of abortions happen after twenty-one weeks), that surgical and medical abortion are not safe (nope, very safe) – and you have a powerful political force. Abortion is rarely about abortion in politics: abortion is politicised to capture all of the ills in society – sex, migration, poor mothers, secular society, poverty, even crime – that clash with the good, old-fashioned values of a time when these ills allegedly didn't exist.

A third explanation for why abortion is such a powerful political tool in contemporary *global* politics is a toxic mix of populism, religion, colonialism and the fear of the foreign other. Political leaders use the language and sentiment of anti-colonialism or anti-imperialism to frame abortion as a threat to the population and a particular way of life. They say abortion is a foreign idea, paid for with foreign money, which is used to change a country's way of life and kill off its population, and therefore something to be resisted. This is a classic political tactic, usually reserved for authoritarian regimes, who use the threat of the outsider to double-down on their repressive politics.

The framing of abortion as a foreign threat to a country is particularly effective because colonialists and imperialists *did* use population control as a means of exerting power over the colonised. Colonial history *is* wrapped up with global health and foreign aid. Women's sexual and reproductive health and control of women's bodies *has* always been a part and parcel of colonialism, either through the export of Western medicine and ideas around birth control and family planning or deliberate sterilisation practices. Forced sterilisation of people living in colonised lands was not uncommon, and in some countries, such as Australia and Canada, was a key part of the settler colonial project. As the next chapter will show, control of women's bodies and reproduction persists in occupied territories such as Palestine. Colonial expansion would not have been possible without medicine and scientific discovery. And, in turn, colonisers brought a range of new health issues and diseases to the people living in the lands they stole.

The supposed risk of malign foreign influence that politicians like to warn about connects with people: first, because, even decades after independence for many ex-colonies, the international health system has not fully acknowledged or redressed the impact of colonialism on sexual and reproductive health, and ex-colonisers prefer a revisionist history of the 'benefits' of empire rather than a frank reckoning with the past; and second, because of the continued presence of international actors in aid-dependent countries. Even if not always malign, foreign influence is not made up. It is there for all to see in the Toyota Land Cruisers covered in 'Save the Girl Child' logos outside the best eateries; the large saving-mothers budgets of ministries of finance and health; and the way in which countries align their priorities to the latest UN development goal or initiative on women's reproductive health. This creates a complex situation and a compelling argument. The leaders who make claims about abortion being part of malign foreign influence are your usual groupings of right-wing politicians, evangelicals, social media influencers and religious leaders. Some of these politicians may care deeply about preventing abortion (though if so they would engage in effective measures to reduce abortion outlined above), but what they all care about is power and drawing on two powerful, evocative issues – family values and colonialism – to gain power. While these leaders tend to be from the country where they seek to influence abortion policy, a large proportion receive funds from abroad, most notably from the US.

Take the example of Malawi. The Malawian government has been trying to reform abortion law and pass the Termination of Pregnancy Bill since 2016. The bill would overturn Malawi's strict ban on abortions to permit it where there is a threat to a woman's physical or mental health, in cases of rape and incest or where there are serious foetal abnormalities. Some politicians and civil servants have been keen to support the bill to uphold their regional commitments to the 2003 Maputo Protocol on the Rights of Women in Africa, and for the plain fact that Malawi has some of the highest rates of maternal mortality in the world, partly due to two-thirds of the country's estimated 141,000 abortions a year ending in complications and the need for post-abortion care.[10] In 2021, the bill came the closest it ever had to passing. Key politicians and community leaders had talked to religious leaders to see if they could reach a common ground.[11] Activists within the movement had a targeted and wide-reaching campaign across the country. And the high-profile death of a fourteen-year-old child following an unsafe abortion shocked Malawians.[12] Yet, still the bill did not pass. As organised as the coalition had been, it did not break the power of the religious right in the country.

Archbishop Thomas Luke Msusa was one religious leader who opposed the bill. Speaking at a World Congress of Families conference entitled 'The African Family and Cultural Colonization' in November 2017, Archbishop Thomas Luke Msusa condemned an earlier version of the bill, noting 'in particular that there are some worrisome trends in our democratization and emancipation that push for a worldview independent of and side-lining God'.[13] For Msusa – like many other leaders of religious organisations such as the Episcopal Conference of Malawi, Muslim Association of Malawi, and Evangelical Association of Malawi – the Termination of Pregnancy Bill went against God's will, and most importantly was linked to a pernicious form of foreign influence on Malawi.[14]

The irony in this is that there was already a pernicious foreign influence in Malawi, and it was paying for the conference at which Msusa was speaking. The World Congress of Families is part of the US-based organisation, International Organization for the Family, which opposes same-sex marriage, the rights of trans and gender non-conforming people and abortion. It was founded in 1997 and specifically targets partnerships in sub-Saharan Africa.[15] A key part of the Congress's strategy is to frame issues of LGBTQ+ rights and abortion as a foreign, colonial other that is being imposed on Africans and African ways of life, drawing vague but convincing links with past colonialism. Abortion is at the front line of this.

The growth of the anti-colonial, populist, right-wing mix has not come out of the blue. As Elżbieta Korolczuk and Agnieszka Graff have shown in their research, it is a deliberate rhetoric and tactic funded by far-right organisations such as CitizenGO, the European Family Foundation and the Alliance Defending Freedom from the US, Germany and Spain, as a means to spread their anti-abortion, anti-women's-rights agenda in other countries. Political, religious and social leaders in these countries accept their money and adopt their rhetoric as a means to access and sustain power. This is another way women's health is used to exert ideological influence – through private finance and philanthropy – and the other is through government policy, such as the global gag rule.

Activists in Malawi were clear that part of the reason the Termination of Pregnancy Bill got stuck was that even those in government who were pro-reform didn't want to upset the US and risk losing out on foreign aid. The campaign to change Malawi's abortion law was happening under Trump's brand of the global gag rule, which resulted in aid cuts throughout the world.[16] If 24 per cent of your gross national income is foreign aid, and between 2017 and 2019 you received $125 million from the US government in aid, you understandably don't want to risk annoying the US president.[17] Despite Trump leaving power in 2021, the fear of the global gag rule and its silencing impact on politicians in countries like Malawi never went away.

The ultimate goal of sexual and reproductive justice activists is to stop the global gag rule in its current form, and then to stop it for good; to end the back and forth. To do this requires allies across the floor within the US Congress putting restrictions on the abortion memos of presidents. You would think that an issue as divisive as abortion would make this impossible. But according to some reproductive justice campaigners, not so. Trump's extension of the global gag rule and his wider attitudes to the office of president led to doors opening in Washington that had been previously shut. Even Republicans would, at times, acknowledge and respond to the evidence of the impact of the global gag rule: that it was not stopping abortions from happening, it was instead threatening the lives and livelihoods of women around the world. And more than that, it was undermining US projects abroad and damaging the reputation of the country.

In 2019, there was hope for change in Congress with the Global Health, Empowerment and Rights Act. This new act planned to establish:

> that a foreign nongovernmental organization shall not be disqualified from receiving certain U.S. international development assistance solely because the organization provides medical services using non U.S. government funds if the medical services are legal in both the United States and the country in which they are being provided. Such foreign organizations shall not be subject to requirements relating to their use of non-U.S. funds for advocacy or lobbying activities, other than those that apply to U.S. nongovernmental organizations.[18]

Sponsored in the Senate by Democratic Senator Jeanne Shaheen and in the House of Representatives by Democratic Representative Barbara Lee, and backed by Kamala Harris, the bill had support across the aisle. The bill was sent to the Senate on 2 July 2019. But as of autumn 2023, the bill was stuck in the system. For bills to become law, both chambers have to pass identical versions of the bill (each chamber can pass different versions, but then they have to meet, reconcile the differences between the two and then agree and pass the bill), which is then subject to sign-off from the president. A colleague clarified all of this to me as I was trying to recall Government 101 from my student days: 'If you suspect the system was designed not to make passing legislation easy, you may be onto something.'

The bigger problem is the timing of the bill. The draft summary states, 'if the medical services are legal in ... the United States'. The idea is that US domestic and foreign policies should align, or, in other words, America should do unto others as it would do unto itself. In 2019, when the bill was drafted, abortion was legal in the US. However, in 2022 this ruling was overturned by the 24 June Supreme Court ruling Dobbs vs Jackson Women's Health Organization et al. Dobbs removed the constitutional right to abortion in the US, meaning that individual states could set their own limits or bans on abortion. As of 2023, fourteen states in the US made abortion illegal, and ten other states introduced strict limits on abortion. Dobbs causes a whole host of complications for the Global Health, Empowerment and Rights Act and how it would be interpreted should a president want to gag the world again. Dobbs also posed an energy problem for activists and politicians. Reproductive justice activists were now fighting a war on three fronts: first, at the federal level with the Supreme Court ruling; second, at the state level to ensure legal protections in states where abortion was still legal and ensure that there was no over-implementation of Dobbs in states where it was restricted; and third, at the international level, where there is always the threat of the return of the global gag rule.

The global gag rule is one of the biggest warning signs women's health activists had had regarding the fragility of Roe vs Wade. Republicans had been attacking these rights all along, but they had been targeting women who lived abroad. When Republicans and far-right movements in the US could not gain traction for overturning abortion rights within the US, they focused on the rest of the world. The global gag rule was part of a right-wing American political movement that started with its focus on other countries in the world and then built momentum working from the outside in, from foreign to domestic policy. As the global gag rule expanded to cover more institutions and countries in the world, so did the domestic pressure to overturn American women's constitutional right to abortion. This was no mistake: the same organisations funding anti-abortion activism and legislation in Europe, Latin America and Africa were often funding anti-abortion legislation in key states in the US, such as Mississippi, and anti-abortion politicians throughout the country. The far-right movement to curtail abortion rights and women's health was always connected between the global and the local.

For decades, poorer countries in the global south have been looking to richer countries in the global north to spot political trends and issues, such as whether a newly elected leader wants to cut aid/trade/diplomatic relations with other countries, or in the realm of women's health, such as whether politicians are pursuing increased support for abortion, contraception and sex education domestically. Sexual and reproductive justice activists in countries such as Malawi were looking at what was happening on abortion in countries such as the US. Had America looked at what the US government was doing in the rest of the world, the warning signs were all there.

Women's health and reproductive justice organisations from around the world want an apology for the harm done to women on account of the global gag rule, and its extension under Trump. The greatest apology of all would be to ensure this never happens again. Women don't have to die because America sneezes its politics into the world. But this sneeze works both ways. Women's health and abortion is an issue that unites US foreign and domestic policy, American women and the rest of the world. Foreign and domestic policy are united in appealing to an electoral base, using the restriction of women's health as a tool of hard power.

Four years on from Trump and the white men in suits that opened this chapter, another president in another January signed another executive order. One of the first acts of Joe Biden when he became president in 2021, like Barack Obama before him and Bill Clinton before *him*, was to rescind the global gag rule. Eight days after his inauguration, Joe Biden issued a memo 'on Protecting Women's Health at Home and Abroad', stating, 'It is the policy of my Administration to support women's and girls' sexual and reproductive health and rights in the United States, as well as globally', and instructing all agencies to immediately reinstate funding to all organisations affected by the gag.[19] He noted the expansion of the gag under Trump and the harmful impact it had had around the world. Biden could stop the global gag rule as a presidential order, but he would not be able stop the Supreme Court from overturning Roe vs Wade and ending the constitutional right to abortion in America.

The US government is known for imposing its interests on the world. The most common understanding of how the US exerts influence is through hard power: of wars, regime change and economic sanctions. The global gag rule demonstrates another means of doing this: through health, and not any health, but women's health. There is one big difference between women's health and other tools of US hard power and foreign policy such as war. Wars in Iraq and Afghanistan (and Vietnam and Nicaragua before that) failed, in part at least because they did not have the support of the people or governments of those countries. Gagging people on women's health works because of the complicity of other governments, other people and the impact of right-wing US private interests and charitable giving of substantial financial aid to these countries. This suggests that all aid-recipient governments are stooges of the US, but this is both simplistic and overlooks the considerable agency these states can have. Aid dependency is only part of the story. The other part is that, as it is for Republican US governments, gagging talk on sexual and reproductive rights is politically attractive to other world leaders.

What gives women's health such power is that it is overlooked as a tool of hard power and foreign policy. This is what makes the global gag rule so effective – it is dismissed as 'just' an issue about women's health or foreign aid spending. It is not something worthy of attention in the way that other aspects of US hard power and coercion are, such as war and economic sanctions. No country has broken a trade deal, a special relationship or sanctioned countries for how they control women's health. They either offer a bit of extra money to fix the problem, do nothing, turn a blind eye or they join in. This is despite the major impact it has on the lives of women and societies throughout the world.

4

Checkpoints, Blockades, Bombs and Pregnant Women

As soon as Amina felt the first pangs of labour, she told her husband that they needed to get in the car and go to hospital. Her maternity hospital was in East Jerusalem, twenty-five kilometres away from her home in Ramallah, in the West Bank of Palestine. She knew the checkpoint that controlled the border wall between home and the hospital could have delays, with queues of traffic backed up along browning grey concrete overseen by security cameras and Israel Defense Forces (IDF) guards. She was not taking her chances. They got in the family Audi and started to make their way to the hospital at the top of a hill in East Jerusalem, an area of Palestine under Israeli control. As Palestinians, they would need permission to enter Jerusalem to get to the hospital. They had their paperwork ready.

Amina's labour was progressing quickly. The traffic leading up to the wall was not. The queue to the checkpoint was long and at a standstill. Closed in, between an orange plastic barrier to her left, heavy concrete barriers to her right, masses of barbed wire leading up the bleak wall and cars all around her, Amina gave birth to her son in the back of the car. Her son would first see her, then people who stopped to help her, the Red Crescent ambulance that had been called, and finally the turret of the Qalandya checkpoint with IDF soldiers looking on under the Israeli flag. Her son's birth certificate noted the place of birth as the 'Qalandya Check Point Behind the Apartheid Separation Wall (Audi A4 Car)'.[1]

Amina is not an anomaly. In 2008, the issue of Palestinian women giving birth at Israeli checkpoints had become so acute that the UN investigated and reported back to the Human Rights Council, the biggest human-rights authority in the world, detailing nine serious concerns with what was happening.[2] The report was part of the growing concern about maternal healthcare in the Occupied Palestinian Territories (OPT) of the West Bank and Gaza Strip, where the reproductive choices of women like Amina were controlled by Israeli permits, checkpoints, border crossings and ever-shifting rules and requirements.

The control of women's access to maternity services in the OPT was not the result of a series of unintended consequences from living under Israeli occupation. It was a form of intentional political control, where women's health becomes a central part of a conflict: something to be curtailed, controlled or, in extreme cases of war, destroyed. This happens in occupied territories such as Palestine, but also in hot conflict zones where access to health facilities is deliberately restricted as a weapon of war. In this chapter, I'm exploring how women's health, particularly maternal health, becomes a target in one of the hardest forms of international politics: war, disputes and conflict. I begin by looking at the long, slow burn on control and curtailment in Palestine (prior to the 2023 conflict, which is happening as I write), before focusing on more short-term, immediate efforts to target and destroy maternal health services in hot conflicts such as Syria and Ukraine. These cases are united by an effort to control, curtail or destroy women's health services by one side of a dispute in order to defeat the other. It is one of the most extreme ways in which women's health can be exploited for political gain.

The choices you face as a pregnant woman like Amina living in the West Bank are impossible. If you opt for a vaginal birth, you wait for labour to begin and then travel to a health facility to give birth. If you make it to a facility run by the Palestinian Authority, chances are you will be in a hospital suffering from under-staffing and overcrowding. That's if you make it to a facility. You know that reaching a health facility is far from simple on account of roadblocks, checkpoints and the 440-kilometre wall. You may be delayed and, as happened to Amina, give birth in your car or at a checkpoint. So instead you think about giving birth at home. Much better than your car. However, what if something goes wrong? Home births are safe and a preferred option for many pregnant people. Most people who decide to have home births do so confident that if something goes wrong they can be blue lit to emergency care. But what if you can't access the emergency care quickly enough because you're probably going to get delayed on your way to the hospital by a checkpoint? If you have family or friends living near a health facility you move in with them. This means, unlike Amina, you probably won't have the support of your partner and immediate family when you give birth, but even so it is highly unlikely they would be able to travel with you anyway. The final alternative is to plan the time and location of your birth: you opt for an elective C-section. Safe, but not without risk. Health researchers in the region noted a growth in C-sections among the Palestinian population in the late 2000s, and attribute this to a C-section being one of the only options available to control labour and birth under such restrictions. This is, of course, if pregnant Palestinians can afford to make the choice to travel or pay for health facilities and services outside public hospitals. Most can't.

Imagine the stress of all of this. It is humiliating and distressing. As the UN report on Palestinian women giving birth at Israeli checkpoints notes, 'Palestinian pregnant women and their families live with anxiety and stress, especially during the last period of pregnancy, of not being assured that they will be able to reach a maternity facility and to return home. Transport between the home and the hospital is a constant concern.'[3] Some women use the concept of *hamm* – a combination of feelings of anger, distress, frustration, grief, worry, unease, sorrow and incapacitation – to describe their experience of reproductive health under such circumstances.[4]

If you lived in Gaza these issues multiplied. Gaza was under blockade temporarily since 2005 and permanently since 2007 by Israel, and Egypt since 2014. The full blockade came after Hamas took control of Gaza in 2007. Hamas is designated a terrorist organisation by Israel, the US, UK and European Union, and the blockade was justified as a means of protecting Israel from Hamas. This does not mean all Palestinians living in Gaza support Hamas. Palestinians have not had the opportunity to vote since Hamas won the Palestinian elections in 2006, when Palestinian politics was effectively split into two entities: Gaza controlled by Hamas and the West Bank ruled by Fatah. The lack of elections since 2006 is a complex interplay of Palestinian elites wanting to hold on to power (which some say is more a concern of Fatah than Hamas), suppression of opposition parties by both the Palestinian elite and the Israeli government, international donors wanting free and fair elections but not wanting Hamas to win again, and the persistent problem of Jerusalem – if Palestinians were allowed to vote in a Palestinian election in Jerusalem, Israel would have to accept the city as Palestinian territory. Elections have been promised but always come to nothing because of the above challenges.

Up until 2023, the blockade meant that Israel controlled the land, sea and air of Gaza, and the movement of people, goods and services in and out of the territory, in effect shutting Gaza off from the rest of Palestine (including essential services such as specialised hospitals) and the rest of the world. After Hamas killed 1,400 people and took 220 hostages in Israel on 7 October 2023, Israel immediately responded by intensifying the blockade and imposing absolute limits of water, oil and food entering Gaza, to the extent that three weeks after the Hamas attacks, Gazans were living off three litres of water a day for all their needs, or just one litre if living in UN shelters.[5]

Between 2005 and 2023, Israel controlled two of the checkpoints in and out of Gaza, and Egypt the third. To leave Gaza you needed a permit. The permit had to be sought from Israeli authorities seven to ten days in advance if you needed healthcare, and you only found out if it had been approved one day before the health appointment. The WHO, the independent health organisation of the UN, reported a total of 3,815 'interrogations' of patients requiring permits to cross the wall between 2008 and 2022, twenty-eight patients arrested for seeking healthcare and 64 per cent of health-worker permits through the WHO denied. A third of all permits for regular healthcare travel were denied or delayed between 2016 and 2022.[6] This, if you can believe it, is an improvement on permit approvals, with less than half approved for healthcare purposes in 2016. Even more alarming, due to restrictions on who could or could not have a permit, 43 per cent of children seeking access to healthcare outside Gaza from 2018 and 2022 travelled without a parent.

If you were a pregnant person seeking healthcare within Gaza during the blockade, chances are you'd be stuck with an overburdened health system on the verge of collapse.

According to experts on women's health in Palestine, such as Doaa Hammoudeh, Rita Giacaman, Weeam Hammoudeh and Tiziana Leone, 'Healthcare in the Gaza Strip has been on the brink of collapse mainly due to siege conditions imposed by Israel and Egypt.'[7] Palestinian authorities have no control over basic health needs such as water supply. The Palestinian Ministry of Health paid higher prices for medical goods and supplies than the international benchmark because of the blockade and the problems it caused getting supplies in and out of the territory. Israel banned medical items that could be of 'dual use' to the military, including everyday essentials such as generators, prosthetics and ambulance-calling equipment.[8] In 2019, according to a report from the director general of the WHO, 42 per cent of all categories of essential medicine were 'completely depleted' in Gaza.

In 2020, there was a 43 per cent increase in maternal deaths in Palestine compared to 2019.[9] Of these deaths, 24.3 per cent were COVID-19 related. The damning part was 78 per cent were avoidable. Avoidable deaths of women – loved women, women with families and friends, and a life to live with their new child – giving birth. It would be easy to interpret this increase in maternal mortality as linked to COVID-19 alone. In the US, for example, maternal mortality rates also shockingly increased by 18.4 per cent between 2019 and 2020.[10] However, looking at maternal mortality rates pre-COVID-19 shows an increase prior to 2020. In 2019, the UN reported a 122 per cent increase in maternal mortality between 2017 and 2018 for women living in Gaza. This increase was attributed to an acute shortage of essential medical supplies, in an already depleted health system.[11] The increase was a shock, given attempts by the Palestinian health sector and international community to improve maternal mortality rates in Gaza and the West Bank, and an overall steady decline in maternal mortality rates since 1993 (though they were still high compared to maternal mortality in Israel and the region). Another statistic that illustrates the situation is the maternal mortality rate for Israeli settlers living in the West Bank in 2020. For women living in the same geographical area as Palestinian women, just with different abilities to move freely for work, family and access to healthcare, the rate was nine times lower than for Palestinians living there.[12] All of this was happening *before* the 2023 war, when hospitals in Gaza were bombed, over a million Palestinians displaced and 50,000 pregnant women – 5,500 of whom were due to deliver in the first month of the conflict – faced air strikes and the humanitarian crisis of an intensified blockade with acute water, fuel and food shortages and destroyed infrastructure and homes.

The Israeli government's response to these issues is: nothing to do with us. Since the 1993 Oslo Accords, which sought to bring peaceful co-existence between Israel and Palestine, health provision for Palestinians living in the OPT, including maternal health, has been the responsibility of the Palestinian Authority, not the Israeli government.

Palestinians living in Israel *are* able to access world-class health facilities within the country. Israel is world-renowned for the quality of its comprehensive health system and as a destination for women's fertility treatment and IVF. It is one of the only places in the world that gives public money to support IVF for two successful births for women aged between eighteen and forty-five, and its fertility clinics boast that they match the top five US clinics for quality at a third of the price. Public provision of IVF is in part linked to the country's reputation for advances in medical technology, the importance of the family in Israeli society and the need to increase Jewish birth rates after the devastation of the Holocaust. While Palestinians living in Israel are also covered by the IVF policy, for some, Israel's progressive IVF policy is more about a pronatalist approach to increasing the Israeli birth rates: to increase the Israeli population as a counter to the Palestinian population.

As one Palestinian health leader explained to me, there is no denying the quality of Israeli health services, but they are also a weapon against Palestinians living in Israel who access them: if you don't behave, you lose the access. In accepting high-quality healthcare, you acquiesce to Israel's power: they give you something you need to stay alive, but in accepting it you legitimise the authority that controls and curtails the health and lives of you, your friends, family and country.

The Israeli argument that the Palestinian Authority is responsible for the health of Palestinians – as set out in the 1993 Oslo Accords – would fly perhaps if the Palestinian Authority was responsible for Palestinian territory, rather than the *Occupied* Palestinian Territory of the West Bank and Gaza. The trick is in the name. Under blockade, the movement of goods, services and people in Gaza was controlled by Israel: this includes direct control of medical goods, services and people. This is a form of direct control. Then there is the indirect control. Part of the problem with Palestinian healthcare under blockade has been the understaffing of and over-demand on hospitals and health centres within Gaza and the West Bank. To address this problem, the Palestinian Authority needs funding and revenue, and to retain healthcare workers within the region. What happens in practice is Palestinian healthcare workers cross the wall to work in cities such as Jerusalem where they get greater pay – seemingly a classic brain-drain problem. Usually in these conditions, workers cross borders to be paid more, and return home with greater income, which is taxed and contributes to state finances. However, compounding the problem for the Palestinian Authority's public purse, the tax revenue derived from Palestinians working in Israel is periodically held back by the Israeli government. Under the 1994 Paris Protocol, Israel collects taxes on behalf of the Palestinian Authority but rarely pays the full amount. Israel justifies withholding the full amount as either punishment for the Palestinian Authority's actions – for example, when it successfully got the UN to instruct the International Court of Justice to offer an opinion on the legality of Israel's occupation of Gaza and the West Bank – or the reallocation of this tax to the families of Israelis killed by Palestinians. The Israeli government's consistent justification for doing this has been that Gaza is run by Hamas, a terrorist organisation. But this says little about the rest of Palestine or the politics of people living in Gaza. The consequence of all this for the health system is: no workers + no revenue = no means of paying to develop the health system or attract and retain health workers. What was happening in the OPT before the 2023 war was not a direct, short-term attack on the health system of Palestine by the Israeli authorities, but a slow burn of depletion, of starving the system of resources. Same with women's health and maternity services: there is not a direct attack on these services which you can pinpoint and condemn, but a slow attrition of access and resources.

Whatever the Oslo Accords say, the idea that women's health in Palestine has nothing to do with Israel is nonsense. The problem with women's access to health in Palestine is one of war, blockades, walls, checkpoints and the lack of free movement created and maintained by Israel. Curtailing women's access to health is a tool of political control: at a basic level, it is a way of reminding a population who has power over them, their lives and their reproduction, in order to break their will and create a cumulative wave of stress, or *hamm*. At a more substantive level, before the war began in 2023, it was about playing the long game: restricting basic services and limiting the growth of a population to win a dispute and extend power over a territory and people. For a country like Israel, the long game works in two ways: curtail Palestinian women's access to maternal health services and boost Israeli women's access to world-beating, publicly funded fertility treatments. It is a war of attrition, where the main battleground is women's health. This is one way of using women's health as a target in a conflict – the slow burn of restrictions, rules, blockades, walls, checkpoints and permits. The other, for those countries involved in active conflict and not wanting to play the long game, is to take extreme measures and go to the source: bombing maternity hospitals.

The first thing that catches your eye in journalist Evgeniy Maloletka's photograph of bombed Maternity Hospital No. 3 in Mariupol, Ukraine on 9 March 2022 is not the debris and devastation left by the Russian bomb, or the woman on the stretcher being carried by five men. It is the hot-pink blanket with black dots and a dash of green. It is the sort of joyous blanket you might buy yourself as a pick-me-up if you're having a bad day, or to bring yourself comfort on the day you go into hospital to give birth. The second thing you see in the photo is her: the woman who was in Maternity Hospital No. 3 when the bomb struck. The woman whose baby was stillborn. The woman who died half an hour after her child. Maternity Hospital No. 3 was bombed on 9 March 2022, one month into the Russian invasion of Ukraine, killing three people and injuring seventeen. The pictures of babies and pre- and post-partum mothers being wheeled out of Maternity Hospital No. 3 were a chilling sign of things to come in the war. Russia would apply the tactics of targeting and bombing health facilities, which it honed in Syria, to Ukraine, and it was going to start with women and babies.

Maloletka's picture of the woman on the pink blanket became worldwide news. Leaders around the world condemned the act. French President Emmanuel Macron called it a 'disgraceful act of war' and the EU declared it a war crime. Macron and the EU were right. Dating back to 1864, the Geneva Conventions say that in times of conflict, medical facilities or personnel are not a target. This rule has remained constant every time the Geneva Conventions have been revised and readopted – in 1906, 1929, 1949 and 1977. And with every major conflict, they continue to be ignored. The UN has made repeated calls for countries to stop targeting medical and health facilities. After high-profile attacks in Syria, Afghanistan and Yemen between 2015 and 2016, the UN Security Council passed Resolution 2286, condemning such attacks and reasserting state obligations under international law not to target health and medical facilities. The resolution had little effect. According to one study, in the second half of 2016, the year the resolution was passed, there were 170 attacks on health facilities in Aleppo, Syria alone.[13] Even more troubling, two of the five permanent members of the UN Security Council were responsible for some of the worst assaults: the US was responsible for airstrikes on Kunduz Trauma Centre in Afghanistan, a hospital run by the humanitarian charity Médecins Sans Frontières (MSF), which killed forty-two people and destroyed the hospital; and according to the Safeguarding Health in Conflict Coalition, 'by far the vast majority of strikes on health have been publicly attributed to the Russian and/or Syrian government forces' carrying out attacks on hospitals. By April 2022, two months after the start of the war in Ukraine, there had already been a hundred attacks on health facilities by Russian forces.[14]

Attacks on health facilities can range from direct bombing campaigns, violence and threats against health workers, ambushing ambulances or stopping and/or delaying them at border checkpoints, stealing and looting medicine and medical supplies, to deliberate blockades of medical personnel and equipment getting in and out of an area. The WHO collects data on attacks against health facilities and workers, monitoring reported attacks by type and location, and using a traffic-light system to clarify whether the reports can be verified. This is a helpful resource but it only tells us part of the story. There are glaring omissions in the data. For example, 79 per cent of health facilities were destroyed in Tigray, Ethiopia between 2020 and 2022, and MSF reported an assault on one of their medical teams in the region, which killed three members of staff in June 2021. Yet up until 2022, the WHO had reported no attacks on health workers in the conflict. We don't know *what kinds* of health facility are targeted. For example, we only know if a maternity hospital is a target if it's reported in the media – this is not captured in the data. Another glaring gap is *who* these attacks impact. A victim's gender is missing from over 40 per cent of the reports on attacks on health facilities.[15] As of 2022, there had only been one study by the Swedish Red Cross on whether this violence affects men and women differently, and it concluded that we really don't know much about this.[16] Gender may make men and women more susceptible to certain kinds of violence. For example, men are more likely to be ambulance drivers and therefore exposed to certain types of risk such as checkpoint attacks, border blockages and hijacking. Women are more likely to be community outreach workers so are at greater risk of attacks in the community. This risk was heightened considerably after the CIA used women health workers and a hepatitis B immunisation campaign as cover to gain intelligence on Osama Bin Laden's compound in Abbottabad, Pakistan. Once it became clear that this intelligence had led to the killing of Bin Laden by US Navy SEALs, there was a rise in attacks on community health workers around the world, from Pakistan to Nigeria. But aside from these stories and reports, we really know very little about who the victims are or if attacks on specific types of healthcare facility, notably maternity hospitals, are a deliberate and sustained tactic of war – other than the fact that it keeps happening.

The WHO depends on member countries to report attacks. Given some member countries are behind the attacks – targeting health facilities either in other countries or in opposition territories in their own countries – they are not keen to report them. Expert Larissa Fast calls these attacks on healthcare 'reputational issues'. Countries don't want to be seen to be targeting health facilities, and the WHO does not want to upset countries that do so, as they are also members of and donors to the organisation. The lack of reporting means we can only estimate the number of attacks on health facilities and health workers and the types of facilities they target – for example, if they target maternity hospitals more than other facilities – and therefore the motivations behind them. If we had better data on what was being attacked, we could start to think about why. The what and why are important, as this information can help with prevention and response, and it points to the motivations and tactics of the conflict. For example, if maternity hospitals are targeted, it could be because the perpetrator sees the conflict as a long war, with the killing of women and children as fundamental to their aims to destroy the enemy's future population.

The intent of attacks on health facilities is to break the infrastructure of a country, to disrupt supplies and services of the enemy and to make it impossible for people to remain living in an area. Some attacks are indiscriminate and some specifically target trauma and maternity hospitals. The former you can in part understand (despite it being illegal): the attacks supposedly target soldiers, not civilians. This is what those responsible say – they are pursuing terrorists. But this rarely holds up at the best of times, even less so as an explanation for *targeted* attacks on maternity hospitals. If you hit a maternity hospital you are not targeting terrorists or soldiers; you want to disrupt women's access to safe birth and you want to kill pregnant women and newborn babies.

After the attack on Maternity Hospital No. 3, Russian Foreign Minister Sergey Lavrov followed the targeting-terrorists line, stating (contrary to all press reports) that the hospital 'no longer sheltered patients, but extremists. It had been seized by the Azov battalion and other radicals. All caregivers had been expelled.' This line is not new to the conflict in Ukraine, and had been used time and again by the Russian-backed Assad regime in Syria. First you accuse the opposition of carrying out the attack themselves, and when that doesn't work you shift to accusing the target hospital of harbouring terrorists. When Lavrov's terrorist argument didn't fly, Russia changed its line of defence, stating the images and reports were all Western propaganda and that the woman on the pink blanket was alive and well and teaching under a Russian flag in Mariupol. Whether you believe me or Lavrov, the point here is that an attack on a women's health facility became a major subject of discussion in the first year of the war in Ukraine. Both sides were using this horrendous bombing to different political ends – one to expose the illegality and brutality of Russia's invasion, the other to condemn Western propaganda. Both claims are powerful: targeting of women's health in conflict – particularly the bombing of the most innocent, mothers and babies – connects and promotes outrage with people around the world. During war and conflict the will to save mothers and children becomes even more pronounced in international affairs. While the will to save mothers has been problematic for women (who are depicted as weaker, to be protected, once again only to have value in the world as mothers who reproduce for their country) and for understandings of conflict (mothers also enact violence in conflict as soldiers, drone operators, strategists), for many, motherhood and newborn babies are powerful symbols of strength, resilience and vulnerability in war. Women's health facilities thus become powerful targets in a conflict, a line not to be crossed in international law, a symbol of hope for the future and proof that life goes on even in the midst of war.

Towards the end of 2022, there were two additional assaults on Ukrainian maternity hospitals – the first in Vilniansk, Zaporizhzhia, the second in Kherson. The Kherson Maternity Hospital was bombed one month after Ukrainian forces had recaptured the city. The attack was a clear signal from the Russians that, despite Ukraine recapturing the city, 'We can still kill your women and children.'

The two stories in this chapter are connected by one thing: the control and restriction, in the case of Palestine prior to 2023, or, in the case of Ukraine, the destruction of women's health services as a target in a conflict. The slow burn of women's health services and direct bombing of maternity hospitals are two sides of the same war crime. What is specific to women's health is that it is targeted as the ultimate signal of masculine power – we can harm or control your women and children – against hope during a conflict. Motherhood and women's maternal health, especially during conflict, become inextricably linked to the future of a country: something to be protected, controlled or destroyed, depending on your position. The control, restriction and destruction of women's access to maternal health services puts women's health at the centre of the hardest expression of power and politics: war and the potential destruction of a country. It is the most extreme way women's health is exploited for political gain.

The first part of this book has been about how women's health is exploited as an issue in global politics, from the soft power of healthwashing countries such as Rwanda, and its central role in foreign aid budgets and planning, to the hard power of US foreign policy, and conflict in Europe and the

Middle East. A common thread across these chapters has been the will to save mothers. These stories show that the problem of fixing women's health is far bigger than looking at what is happening in science, health and medicine. The problem is not that women's health is embedded in global politics, but that it is so effective as a political tool. If you want to shift the way foreign aid works, change the domestic policy of another country, get elected or control a population, exploiting women's health will do the job. But this is only part of the story of exploitation. The other part is how women themselves are exploited within the health and foreign aid sector. This is the subject of Part 2.

Part 2

Exploiting Women

5

Selling Trauma

'What are you going to do with your power?' asked the chair of the morning session of the UN's 2019 population conference in Nairobi, Kenya.

'I am going to give up my seat and give it to Sylvie.'

The CEO of a major international charity stood up, unclipped her microphone and walked into the audience. Sylvie, a young woman from South Sudan, took her seat on the main stage in front of an audience of women's health specialists. A mix of civil servants sent by their country delegations, activists and other domestic and international charity workers from around the world sat drinking coffee and eating the free doughnuts as they settled in for another busy day at the UN conference.

As soon as the CEO stood up and walked off, the audience started to applaud. Here was a white woman from a powerful organisation sharing her space and giving this young black woman a seat at the table. The applause was akin to when a musician stops a concert and brings a fan on stage to sing or dance with. A disruption to the usual order of things, choreographed with just the right amount of rehearsed spontaneity.

Sylvie looked nervous. She began to tell her story in a

three-part narrative: the trauma, its impact and how she turned her life around with the help of the international charity. As soon as she finished her story, the CEO joined her back on stage, where an additional chair had been placed. The CEO took the mic and talked about the need to think about humanitarianism in a different way, with girls, young women like Sylvie, and gender at its core. The panel continued with a human-rights defender from Lebanon talking about the vibrant feminist movement in the country, and a representative from the Red Cross reading out a set of talking points on gender as if prepared by his HR department.

As I sat listening to Sylvie's story, I realised something. I had zoned out. At the end of her story I couldn't even remember if it was about FGM, sexual abuse or gender-based violence. I knew it was one of the three, but by the time the talk had progressed to the Q&A I couldn't recall which. This is not because I did not value Sylvie's life, her story or her sharing it. It's because I had heard this kind of story, told in this way, many times before. The stories had started to blur into one. The three-part narrative of trauma to hope becomes a well-trodden script. As soon as the script is finished, the storyteller is silent. I was guilty of the type of lack of engagement Susan Sontag warned about in her book on images of conflict, *Regarding the Pain of Others*, where she notes that some people – me – have the privilege of looking away and engaging in 'the cliché of the cosmopolitan discussion of images of atrocity to assume that they have little effect'.[1] Justifying looking away because you've heard the story before, and been saturated with images, is part of the problem. For Sontag, when people feel safe, they feel indifferent. Perhaps I was guilty of such privileged indifference, sat there safely with my coffee and doughnut, but I was also conscious of something else at play. After Sylvie had told her story she was silent. No one asked her a question, she did not respond to any general questions in the Q&A, she did not go off script, and I had no idea what would happen to her after she finished. Like the kid dancing on stage with the pop star at a concert, her participation had been rehearsed, she had her moment in the spotlight, and then it went back to the more powerful woman being the centre of attention.

The other reason I don't recall Sylvie's story is because I was busy watching the audience lap it up. They wanted Sylvie's story and wanted to believe in her empowerment. Sylvie was not asking to be saved; she was saving herself. She was using the attention to empower herself and others around her. Not, supposedly, to empower the major charity that had paid for her to be there, or their fundraising campaign.

What happened with Sylvie and the panel is a new version of an old tactic: the selling of women's trauma as a means of eliciting an emotional reaction in the audience so they act on the wider issue. The action is usually giving money to a cause, to help women like Sylvie and those organisations that support them. It is an old tool of the humanitarian and anti-poverty sector, and it is increasingly common in the health sector. You may be familiar with it. The leaflets that come through your door, the faces that look out at you on the sidebar of the news website you're reading, the big fundraisers who centre such stories and have a link you can click to donate a certain sum to save a life. Look at those pictures. Chances are they are a woman, girl or boy, most likely with black or brown skin. They are rarely a man, and never a white man. Perhaps with good reason: these images represent the recipients of aid money. But ask yourself what they represent about the person, the country they live in, the charity, and the setting or context. What is problematic about these images is how the women in them are often defined by their trauma – whether they are still in need of help or have already been empowered – and the context in which these pictures are taken. The unsettling part is not just the use of such stories, but the fact that women and girls are approached for their stories when they seek out healthcare; and that it is the very organisations who are supposed to help vulnerable women and girls access health who are doing the exploitation.

For feminist scholars such as Akanksha Mehta and bell hooks, what happened in the conference room may have been the creation of a space where some eat the trauma of the other. Where the experience and ethnicity of women like Sylvie 'became spice'.[2] In the past, we ate the trauma of other women to feel bad and to raise money to help them. Women's stories were once told by international charities *for* them, whereas now the expectation is women themselves tell their own stories. Now we eat the trauma of other women's health as a means of empowering or ceding space to these women. The intent has shifted to giving them a voice, visibility and a seat at the table to showcase how representative and inclusive we are. For some women, the act of taking up space and telling your story is an important empowerment tool. And we need different voices in the world to help understand our diverse and ever-changing world and challenge our preconceptions and ideas. But when you cut through Sylvie's story, other than the fact she was telling it, the narrative arc was the same. She had to tell a deeply personal tale about her own trauma and health to get people to take her needs seriously.

The selling of trauma stories is prevalent in fundraising in the aid and health sector because such individual stories are seen to resonate and connect with people. If you have an issue you care about, say cervical cancer, it is not enough to say that cervical cancer kills 342,000 people a year, and is the fourth most common cancer among women.[3] Lots of cancers kill people every year. Cervical cancer is competing with a whole range of other cancers and health issues to attract attention for research investment, funding for palliative care and treatment to support people affected. On top of that, cervical cancer is not only competing for attention in the health space; health in turn has to compete with a range of other societal needs, wants and, in some cases, evils such as rape and abuse to gain the attention and money of people and politicians. To stand out against these competing needs, wants and evils, to elevate the issue of cervical cancer, you have to frame it in a certain way. Issue framing can start with simple numbers – how many people are affected or, the classic, lives saved – but often this does not cut through with politicians or the public. What you need is a story to sell. One with the right amount of trauma and redemption.

A personal story is meant to cut through the numbers of 342,000 people affected by cervical cancer and personalise it. You can't feel sorry for the number 342,000, but you can feel sorry for Sara, who looks like your sister, or a young woman like Sylvie, standing on a stage in front of you. The more personal, the better. One film-maker who worked in the charity sector told me of the key target audience for such stories: Claire, a white woman in her mid-thirties who lives in north London and reads the *Guardian* for news and the *Daily Mail* for celebrity gossip. You may have a similar reaction to mine: am I Claire? If you can't walk past a chugger (charity mugger, the people who stand on busy streets getting you to sign up to give money to charity) without them stopping you, repeatedly (my personal best is three in a row on the same Islington street – as north London as you can get), then yes, you are Claire.

The story and its target audience rests on the notion that Claires can save Sylvies. Both Claire and Sylvie are being exploited in this situation: Sylvie the young woman, or often girl, of colour whose trauma is being eaten by the viewer, and Claire who is regularly stopped on the street and asked for their money. It is another trope of women saving women, and at its worst is set up to propagate white saviourism.

Women can't just be sick or a victim of trauma. To get someone to help us we have to relive and narrate our trauma, and it happens again and again. Fundraising and agenda setting for various health issues depend on women like Sylvie telling these stories. Men do not have to do this. Rarely do you see personal stories of men being used to justify fundraising or political attention for a specific health issue. It is not Carl from north London who is constantly being stopped on the street to save Steve. These stories and images are always of women, mostly young women, and children. As we saw in Part 1, women – especially mothers – who are vulnerable to deadly diseases are seen in the aid world as worthy of help and assistance. This is obviously a dangerous gender stereotype that cuts both ways: men are also vulnerable and worthy of help, and women are not completely devoid of agency. Then there is the Claire and Sylvie principle: women give to more charitable organisations (men give to fewer, but give more money, though women give more when they are paid more), so the assumption is women will give to other women, especially if both women are mothers. With the exception of the early HIV/AIDS crisis in the 1980s, where men and women both publicly shared their stories and engaged in acts of civil disobedience and direct action, it is rare that men have to perform or sell their stories to get their health taken seriously. More than that, the whole fundraising and marketing strategy of major international charities does not rest on men's stories and their willingness to tell them again and again on various platforms: it rests on young women and girls. This works for all international charities, not just health ones.

What is particular about health and medical charities is how they obtain their stories. The issue of eating trauma becomes thornier when questions arise as to who owns these stories, who controls how they are used and where they end up. This is where eating and selling trauma shifts from a white saviour irritant to a serious safeguarding problem for young women and girls. What is worse is that it is not politicians or companies benefiting from such lapses in protection: it is major medical charities.

In 2021, a teenage girl living in Ituri Province in the northeast of the Democratic Republic of Congo (DRC) sought help from a clinic run by the medical humanitarian charity Médecins Sans Frontières (MSF) after a major sexual assault. Doctors treated her for her injuries and gave her medication to prevent HIV, in case she had been exposed to the virus. Once she was settled, she was approached by a photographer working for the organisation. She was asked to share her story and be photographed. She agreed. The pictures were taken metres away from the health clinic where she sought help. They were subsequently used in marketing materials for MSF: the story of how she was a survivor of gang rape, with a photograph of her face alongside it.

The teenager was exactly the subject the photographer commissioned by MSF was looking for. She had a terrible story of sexual violence, remedied by the healthcare provided by the charity. It didn't matter that she was a minor; the photographer received no instruction not to take pictures of children. Children, especially young girls, connect more with viewers when you are trying to galvanise action on an issue, or maybe to win a photography award. As the photographer explained when asked, the girl 'is not a typical 16 year old ... no, she lives in East Congo, in an area where rape is an instrument of war.'

In 2022 you could buy this photograph of 'not a typical' girl, a survivor of sexual violence, for £375 via a stock image library.

Stock images are used for all sorts of reasons: to illustrate publications, news articles, reports, websites, campaigns, strategy documents, fundraising initiatives and countless other possibilities. Some sites offer images for free, others charge. If you type MSF into a major image library such as Getty Images, two types of picture dominate: the first is white doctors with MSF tabards vaccinating black children, the second an anonymous, blue-gloved hand holding out a thermometer gun to the side of a black or brown child's face. Sometimes the child is smiling, sometimes they are grimacing. And then there are the 1,900 images of vulnerable people like the teenager: girls seeking healthcare after 'being gang raped at gun point', children covered in scabs and flies, naked and/ or semi-conscious children. Almost all of these children are Black or brown. All available for you to buy.

We don't know how many of these images of vulnerable women, girls and boys exist. Benjamin Chesterton of the production company duckrabbit, an expert in the use of images in humanitarian settings, explained to me that a photographer may take over five thousand pictures on one shoot. Images of vulnerable people available to buy could number in the hundreds of thousands rather than tens of thousands. Chesterton has been tracking the images available on stock websites such as Magnum Photos for years and sees what happened with this particular MSF image as part of a wider problem of 'humanitarian' photojournalism being normalised child abuse.[4] For him, the problem is not incompetence or lack of awareness, but profiteering from all involved – the photographers, the charities that instruct them and those who reward this work through high-profile awards and repeat contracts. He describes the whole business of humanitarian photojournalism as acting 'like cowboys' and says that these issues are 'rife through an industry that is fundamentally racist and dangerous'.

MSF did not, and in some cases, could not, stop the sale of these photographs and has been clear that the organisation does not profit from the sale of these images from stock agencies. The organisation may commission a photographer to take the pictures but, according to their contract, once a specific time period passes, the photographer owns the copyright and can choose what to do with the images, including selling them. However, not owning the copyright to these images does not let organisations such as MSF off the hook: they commission the images in the first place, and they can set contractual parameters on who is in the pictures and how these pictures are used. The problem is, up until 2022, they didn't. This is in an organisation that works in seventy-two countries and, at last count in 2021, had had one million people stay in their hospitals and had performed 12.6 million consultations.[5] MSF has a reputation for working with some of the most vulnerable people in the world, from Syria to Yemen. But until 2022 – when campaigners started to create noise around the issue – the organisation had no safeguarding policy on the use of images.

We don't know who buys them. We don't know who would want to own an image of a survivor of sexual violence or of a naked, semi-conscious child. Or perhaps we do, but don't want to think about it.

In May 2022, Chesterton, alongside a group of former MSF employees, photographers, film-makers, academics and artists, organised an open letter to the international president of MSF about MSF images available to buy, noting some 'are so disturbing we chose not to list them here'.[6] The open letter sought answers to four key questions:

1. How is it possible that a fully identifiable photograph of a 16 year old child, gang raped at gunpoint, seeking medical help from MSF, ends up published in marketing materials?

2. What happens to these images of vulnerable children that are taken in the clinics you staff?
3. Did the children's parents give informed consent?
4. Do MSF's western staff apply a different set of ethical standards and legal protections to the patients they treat overseas than the patients they treat at home?

The open letter was covered in the *Guardian* and trended on social media.[7] The international president of MSF and the organisation's director of communications provided swift responses. They acknowledged and apologised for the mistake in publishing such images, and committed to accelerating a range of new measures and initiatives the organisation was already undertaking. These measures included a review of the MSF image archive for sensitive images; 'reaching out' to photographers who owned the copyright to the images; reviewing contracting and licensing procedures under the 'do no harm' principle; reviewing content production guidelines; strengthening training and development of content producers; and thinking through best practices for informed consent.[8] All appropriate measures that you may have assumed the organisation was already taking.

The statements from MSF did not directly respond to the four questions in the open letter. The explanation seemed to be that in one case the girl did give informed consent and was supported in doing so. The bigger issue is that at the time the scandal broke, MSF did not own the copyright and therefore the control of how the images are used. Such control and copyright was held by the photographer. The fourth question went completely unaddressed.

MSF's statement does not address what it means to give informed consent in a humanitarian crisis. According to Chesterton, people in these images make a 'devil's bargain'. Whatever they're told, they are participating in the photographs because they think some benefit will come from doing so. This is not full consent; it is an asymmetrical power relation where someone does something because the person asking them has power. This is bad enough if the person participating is an adult, and is definitely not full consent if they are children. As Chesterton put it to me, there is a reason children cannot give informed consent. In addition to the asymmetries of power and the fact that naked pictures of child abuse survivors should not be taken and sold on image websites, a child does not know what they are consenting to. Your young child may consent to run across the street to see their friend, but you are not going to let them do it as you know the risks. The point is no adult should be asking a child to run across the street in the first place, let alone sell their trauma to fundraise for a medical charity.

Ask anyone who has ever sat on or applied to a university ethics committee: some things are universal, including the fact that minors cannot give informed consent. Their parents can on their behalf, but even then, special measures have to be put into practice to ensure no harm can come to the minor or the parent and that both are fully aware of the potential immediate and long-term consequences of their participation. I have some experience of this. I made a film about women living with HIV/AIDS and had to think about all these issues throughout the process. I went back and forth on the inclusion of children and the consent of their parents. To cut a long story short, children were included in the film but their inclusion was tightly controlled. It was controlled by their parents, the cast of the film, me and the ethics department of my university, and was an ongoing conversation throughout the project. I don't know if I got this right. But I do know the children themselves were not in a position to consent. If there isn't parental consent, and if there aren't limits on their participation, then no children can be allowed. Basic ethics. Basic safeguarding.

When campaigners scratched further, they saw myriad

problems with the safeguarding practices of medical human-itarian organisations. Ex-MSF employee, sexual exploitation and abuse activist and co-signatory of the MSF letter, Monica Mukerjee realised staff had little knowledge of 'basic protec-tion standards, working with survivors of violence, and even understandings of what violence is' when she worked for the medical charity. For her, despite MSF's commitment to 'bear witness' to the suffering of vulnerable populations, it had failed to take meaningful action to safeguard the rights of its patients or to enforce disciplinary measures when they were breached. One big example of this has been the failure of MSF to introduce a charter of patients' rights, which would give standard protections to patients and provide the basis for ac-countability of MSF to the people who use the organisation's services.

Doctors working for MSF – rather than the marketing and fundraising teams who commission and organise the stories – had a form of cognitive dissonance about what was happening in the marketing part of the organisation. Or, as organiser of the letter to MSF, Chesterton, describes it, they 'don't want to see how the sausage is made'. Health staff resent the marketing side of their work, but accept it as a necessary evil in order to secure the funds to do the work they do. If this seems a bit of a cop out, it is. While not responsible for commissioning, taking or storing the pictures, they are still in the health setting where it happens. They could still speak out (and many have, given the letter). The problem is the wider culture of organisations such as MSF, where people know what goes on, and either want to speak out but are concerned about what happens if they do, or don't speak out. Neither suggests an organisation where protection of the most vulnerable is the priority.

There is an easy solution to this exploitation. Stop taking pictures of vulnerable women and young girls, stop using these images in marketing and fundraising strategies and stop allowing these images to be sold to third parties. If you can't stop with all vulnerable women, at least draw the line at minors. No children. More than that, the onus is on the photographer to prove the person in the photograph is not a child.

There is a reason these images persist and women keep on telling their stories. Audience. We consume them. If we did not click on the image, buy the print, stop in our tracks when we heard a story, then they would stop. The other issue is, as Susan Sontag cautioned, we've become inured to tragedy. Another disease, another war, another crisis. Attention has to be grabbed by pushing extremes. The problem is the consumer, not the provider. We need to demand better as consumers, storytellers and content providers. If someone wants to tell us their story, we need to be clear on how it will be used and how we benefit. We need to demand better consent and representation practices of the stories we engage with. This could be as simple as not giving money/clicking on links/ liking images of children or trauma, or creating and watching more thoughtful, representative types of storytelling. Or, as I suggest in the Epilogue, taking more direct action by checking the safeguarding policies of major medical humanitarian charities and writing to them/your political representative to ensure these are up to date and being followed.

However, in the case of MSF, Mukerjee and Chesterton are not buying this audience-demand argument. They see it as 'post-rationalising'. The role of the audience only became a part of the argument once MSF were exposed and all other arguments – bearing witness, the child in the picture wanted them to take it, recording history – had run dry. It is insulting to the people who support MSF. I've always liked MSF and seen first hand the incredible work the charity does. When I was in Sierra Leone during the Ebola outbreak, when much of the international community cleared out of West Africa

during the crisis, MSF was one of the handful of organisations that stayed. The more I look into health crises around
the world, the more often MSF is there, staying behind when
everyone else leaves – and so I find it hugely disheartening that
the organisation is in the selling-trauma-of-minors-for-money
game. There are alternative ways of capturing and showcasing
humanitarian crises without demeaning, dehumanising and
exploiting the people in the pictures, from the use of cartoon
or graphic storytelling, using trained actors from the region to
represent the story, to co-production of how the story is told
by adults who want to tell. Storytelling does not have to fixate
on trauma or the bad thing that happened to someone: this
can be a part of a story, but not the sole story of a person's
life, community or healthcare setting. Shifting the blame to
the audience, the Claires of this world, is just another way
of dodging responsibility and accountability for exploitative
practices.

Women and girls can only get the world to take their health
needs seriously if they have a traumatic story that connects
with audiences and can be monetised. Not only is this depress-
ing in itself, it also creates a set of hierarchies. Women have
to be the right kind of victim – young, vulnerable, photogenic
and able to tell a coherent narrative. This not only exploits
women and their trauma, but reinforces the idea that it is
women we should be saving and helping, not men. In addition,
stories of trauma have to be more and more extreme to attract
attention. There is a trauma race to the bottom that leads
those who are supposed to help women access healthcare to
go to greater extremes in how they support this.

   This exploitation is not being enacted by the usual suspects
we think of when we think of the exploitation of women
and health, i.e. right-wing politicians or populist leaders. It
is major international charities and medical humanitarians

doing the exploiting, and it is taking place in health settings and major international health conferences.

The CEOs of charities like MSF are supposed to be the good guys. In 1999, MSF won the Nobel Peace Prize. The good-guys narrative is a problem: it means we turn away from them and assume they are doing the right thing, or we remain silent to protect the rest of the work they do. Such silence in the NGO sector is really bad but, as I show in the next chapter, the consequences are even worse when this happens in the UN.

6

Sexual Exploitation, Abuse, Harassment and the UN

When the first case of Ebola was identified in Mangina, in the North Kivu part of the Democratic Republic of Congo (DRC) on 1 August 2018, the whole community was understandably shocked and scared. People had started to notice friends and neighbours dying but were not sure what was happening. Another Ebola outbreak on the other side of the country in Équateur had been brought under control weeks earlier. Given how far away the Équateur outbreak was, the people of Mangina were hesitant to attribute deaths in the community to a major Ebola outbreak. When patients showed up at the local health centre with diarrhoea, vomiting and fever, doctors and nurses thought patients had malaria. You don't need to wear PPE when treating malaria patients, so several nurses were exposed to the virus. When lab results started to come through, it was clear that what was happening in Mangina was a severe outbreak of Ebola. Ebola is scary because it can spread quickly and goes against every human instinct to care for, hug and touch a loved one. It is even scarier when the spread is happening in a part of the world that is subject to armed conflict. Unlike the 2014/16 Ebola outbreak in Guinea, Liberia and Sierra Leone, this outbreak of Ebola was happening in the conflict hotspot of the DRC. This meant that, in addition to the usual concerns experts like me have about how health emergencies impact on women more than men (health and social care burdens on women, rising levels of domestic violence under lockdowns or curfews, potential increased maternal mortality as women avoid health clinics and the threat of infection for women health workers on the front line), responding to the outbreak had the added complication of having to navigate a conflict with a significant reputation for gender-based violence.

The Ministry of Public Health and the international community moved quickly to address the outbreak. By 2 August, representatives of the health ministry, the WHO, UNICEF and MSF were all in the region to get surveillance systems off the ground to assess how the virus was spreading and whether they were dealing with a new strain. No one could move in or out of a building without washing their hands or having their temperature taken. Contact tracing was mobilised and community leaders were brought in from the outset to educate their communities about how to prevent the spread of Ebola, what to do if someone had Ebola and to help track cases where they lived. North Kivu was awash with chlorine. More international actors arrived. As one nurse from Mangina put it, it was baffling to see such a small town on the world's map: 'This is the first time we have seen the national health minister, the WHO Director-General and the Regional Director for Africa here. Their visit and the start of vaccination for people at risk have kept us in good spirits.'[1]

Unlike the 2014/16 Ebola outbreak, which saw people run away from Ebola, in North Kivu the international community was running towards it. With them came resources: resources to stop Ebola, and resources that support humanitarian efforts as they move around the world – drivers, food budgets, extra personnel, communication equipment and a whole range of ephemera that often contrasts sharply with the wealth and resources available to those living in the region.

By April 2019, eight months after the first identified case, the government of the DRC and the international community were investigating 2,300 Ebola alerts every day, with 3,312 confirmed cases in the country. Despite substantial effort, the international response was not making the progress to get Ebola under control that everyone had hoped for. The WHO – which was co-ordinating the Ebola response alongside the government of the DRC – called for an 'urgent injection' of US$20 million to ensure operational capacity could be sustained well into mid-2020.[2]

As the WHO called for more aid to stop Ebola, another crisis was emerging right under its nose. Reports started to bubble up that women and girls were being sexually abused, harassed and exploited by health workers who were part of the international teams involved in stopping Ebola. Some of these women were working as part of these teams, being asked for sex in exchange for promotion or better pay. Others were young girls who had nothing to do with Ebola or healthcare, raped and exploited by men working for health organisations. The sexual exploitation, abuse and harassment of women and girls by people working to stop Ebola – the very people and organisations that were meant to be helping the community – was so widespread that for many working in the DRC at the time it was an open secret. The more open this secret became, the more senior leaders of the WHO looked away.

Women and girls were exploited twice by the WHO: first, as victims of sexual abuse and exploitation; and second, as survivors whose quest for justice became secondary to efforts to protect the WHO and its senior leadership. The story of women and girls in the DRC is one of women undervalued and exploited in health and health emergency settings, and of members of the international health community who are supposed to help doing harm.

'Jolianne' worked on the side of the main road in Mangina selling top-up credit for phones.[3] Selling phone credit is an essential job in the DRC but not a lucrative one. The injection of a major international presence helps increase the customer base, but not massively. The work usually involves waiting for passing drivers to extend their arm out of the car window with a banknote for the amount of credit they want to buy. Vendors like Jolianne hand over the cardboard vouchers and off the drivers go, either passing the voucher to their boss or scratching the card with one hand while entering the code into their phone with the other. At the end of a long day in April, a driver stopped to buy credit from Jolianne. He offered her a lift home. She agreed. The driver did not take her home. He took her to a hotel and raped her. She later found out she was pregnant.[4]

Jolianne was thirteen. The driver worked for the WHO.

When an independent commission was launched to investigate sexual abuse and exploitation by the WHO during the DRC Ebola outbreak, over fifty women came forward, and Jolianne was one of them. They informed investigators that they were raped, offered work in exchange for sex, told they had to have sex to keep their jobs, and/or offered abortion pills to terminate pregnancies arising from the abuse. While many perpetrators preyed on the young and less educated, like Jolianne, others targeted older professional women. 'Isala', working in the surveillance team, described her experience to the independent commission investigating the abuse and exploitation in the following way: 'Her boss ... told her that she had to give him half her salary or have sex with him to get the job. She paid him for four months, before finally complaining to her superiors. The payments stopped but the doctor was never sanctioned and continued to harass her.'[5]

The perpetrators of the abuse in the DRC were not a handful of bad apples. Abuse and exploitation were systemic in the Ebola response. The independent commission identified eighty-three alleged perpetrators, twenty-one of whom could be directly linked to the WHO. They worked at all levels, as drivers, doctors, service providers, managers, infection control trainers and security officers. They came from all over the world. They were supposed to protect people from harm and represented an organisation that is supposed to be committed to women's health. These were the people who raped, abused and exploited women and girls whose ages ranged from thirteen to forty-two.

The WHO is the leading health agency in the world and is part of the UN. Paula Donovan, a campaigner against sexual exploitation, called what happened 'the biggest finding of sexual abuse perpetrated during a single UN initiative in one area or one country during the time-bound period of a UN response effort'.[6]

The WHO Africa regional director at the time, Matshidiso Moeti, apologised to victims, saying she was 'humbled, horrified, and heartbroken'. In a similar apology, the then director-general of the WHO, Tedros Adhanom Ghebreyesus (commonly referred to by just his first name, Tedros), called the testimonies 'harrowing' and the report a 'dark day' for the institution. As the head of the organisation, he would take full responsibility.

'Dark days', 'zero tolerance', 'thoughts and prayers'. We have heard these words from leaders of UN agencies before. During the 1990s, the UN seemed to be in perpetual crisis over scandals of sexual abuse and exploitation. There were allegations of UN peacekeeper involvement in trafficking women for sex in Bosnia and Herzegovina in the late 1990s; UN staff abusing women and girls in refugee camps in Guinea during the civil war in Sierra Leone; and transactional sex, e.g. sex in exchange for food, shelter and money, between young women and staff from the United Nations Mission in Liberia (UNMIL).[7] In documenting such cases, experts Jasmine-Kim Westendorf and Louise Searle highlighted how cash for sex between peacekeepers and women in countries such as Haiti and East Timor was so prevalent that in East Timor T-shirts were sold with the logo, 'Feel safe tonight, sleep with a Peacekeeper'.

The cascade of abuses that came to light during this period led the then secretary-general of the UN, Kofi Annan, to issue a 'Zero Tolerance' UN bulletin on sexual abuse and exploitation. Annan made clear the obligations of staff under the UN Charter and UN International Civil Service Code of Conduct (in effect since 1954, and revised in 2001 and 2017 – allowing no excuse that zero tolerance was somehow new or out of touch). What followed was a series of taskforces, reports to the UN General Assembly (where all UN member countries meet), and strategies to stop sexual abuse and exploitation among peacekeepers and the wider UN.

For successive secretary-generals, getting rid of the 'scourge' of sexual abuse and exploitation was always something that should go beyond the main corridors of power in the UN in New York, and be taken seriously across the whole organisation. This meant it also had to apply to those UN organisations that did not have a role in international peacekeeping, such as the WHO, a technical, specialised agency within the UN.

The WHO therefore fell under the UN guidelines, training, staff code of conduct and zero-tolerance approach to sexual abuse, exploitation and harassment. The problem with the WHO, as the independent commission investigating what happened in the DRC outlined, is that no one in the WHO followed existing protocols and those that existed were found wanting. No one really did the training. This is perhaps unsurprising: such training is seen as an inconvenience at the best of times, but even more so when you have an Ebola outbreak to deal with. This is a classic tale of the emergency imperative: no one has any time for anything but responding to the crisis itself, regardless of how their actions in a crisis may create additional crises. The lack of concern around these issues in a country such as the DRC, which has some of the highest rates of sexual violence against women in the world, shows an absolute disregard for the context in which the WHO is working. Any DRC expert, women's group, or sexual violence or gender and health expert would tell you that an intervention in the DRC needs sensitivity and awareness around issues of sexual violence and abuse. But no one thought about it and no one thought to ask.

Part of the problem is health crises have historically been seen as something separate from conflict or humanitarian crises. Although health crises can have clear humanitarian effects – they can displace people, disrupt access to food and shelter and make vulnerable people even more vulnerable – they are seen as distinct or different. This may seem a bit of a technical issue, but it is an important one. If two crises are seen differently, for instance an Ebola outbreak and a major earthquake, then the response to them is different. In some ways this makes sense: you do respond to an Ebola outbreak differently than to an earthquake. But some things remain the same: you are dealing with vulnerable people, in unstable, fast-moving contexts, with large injections of cash into the local economy and wrecked infrastructure, and often there is a clear distinction in power between the responders and the vulnerable, in wealth or other needs. Hence, health crises such as an Ebola outbreak come with the same risks as a humanitarian crisis such as an earthquake. Where there are vulnerable people and power imbalances, there is a risk of exploitation and abuse. It is crazy no one thought about this when WHO staff entered the DRC to deal with Ebola. WHO staff may not be peacekeepers, but the same extremes of inequality and vulnerability apply.

There was no effort to prevent sexual abuse and exploitation of women and girls by WHO staff in the DRC, because it was not meant to happen in the health sector. The health sector remains a sacred space of care and concern. Sexual violence and abuse happens among peacekeepers, sure, but that's in the fog of war where sexual violence and rape are weapons of war. This is not the norm in the health sector, and it should definitely not be the norm that health workers themselves are the perpetrators.

Megan Daigle and colleagues explain this as the 'stranger danger' problem – the idea that threats exist out there, some-where else, in foreign countries where aid workers operate, rather than the aid workers themselves being the threat.[8] Daigle reviewed the security manuals and aid worker chat groups, and interviewed key humanitarian workers to see how risks and threats are framed in the humanitarian sector. What she found is the idea that all danger and risk emanated from 'the field' – the country where the foreigner works. All security manuals were written to address this and there was little, if anything, about danger emanating from people you know, the international community, or locals from the country or region who work under the umbrella of an aid charity or UN agency. Young women and girls in the DRC were at risk as no one in the WHO ever thought that they or their colleagues would be the threat.

If the WHO had followed the correct protocol on sexual abuse, exploitation and harassment – establish an identifiable point person in the country with a clear chain of command to senior leaders; mandatory training on how to detect and prevent abuse, exploitation and harassment for *all* employees; set up and communicate ways to report abuse among the community; and investigate, and if necessary report, any claim against an employee – then the senior leaders within the institution *would* have known. If anyone had valued the lives of women working on Ebola, and those in the community in which it happened, the scale and degree of harm being done would have been too important to ignore. It would have constituted something you bother your boss about. Yet, the boss of the WHO at the time – Tedros – swore he only found out about the sexual abuse and exploitation when stories started to appear in the press.

During the period in which workers for the WHO were engaging in sexual exploitation and abuse in the DRC, the Charities Commission of England and Wales published the results of its inquiry into exploitation and abuse in the international charity, Oxfam. The inquiry into Oxfam focused on two issues.[9] The first was the charity's management of allegations against staff working on disaster relief in Haiti in 2010/11. The second was an examination of Oxfam's wider safeguarding measures. It was the Haiti issue that blew up in February 2018, following a report in *The Times* that Oxfam workers had used sex workers on Oxfam property, and the 'women' involved were actually minors. Some staff members had tried to report it to more senior managers and others were being bullied into keeping quiet. The Charities Commission noted reports of allegations and warnings as far back as 2010/11. In November 2010, senior staff were made aware of concerns over poor safeguarding. In July 2011, a whistle-blower raised the issue in an international programme leadership meeting. Concerns did lead to internal investigations of ten staff in

Haiti at the time. However, there was a problem with how this was done. There was a noted 'lapse in good investigations standards' that 'compromised the safety' of witnesses and whistle-blowers. Some of the perpetrators were given a 'dignified exit' or, in other words, a quiet agreement between them and the organisation, and other perpetrators were given a reference from Oxfam with no note on the circumstances under which they had left. Oxfam's defence of the first instance was that the employee was helping the organisation expose further abuse and exploitation, and a dignified exit was a way of enabling this co-operation. On the reference, this was a tricky legal point and Oxfam claimed that this type of reference was accepted as a red flag within the sector. In both cases, the Charities Commission saw this as poor judgement, and found that there was unequal treatment of staff.

The facts remain: abuse and exploitation by Oxfam staff took place on Oxfam property, and despite attempts to notify senior management, some staff were bullied into silence. Even after the claims came to the surface, there were suggestions of a cover-up, or at the very least a lack of transparency as to what was going on.

Once *The Times* report was published, more people came out to talk about the problems of safeguarding within Oxfam. The former head of safeguarding, 2012–15, Helen Evans, was one of the main whistle-blowers. Evans told Channel 4 news in the UK that she was first aware of allegations of this kind in 2013/14, when her team conducted a survey of staff working in the Horn of Africa.[10] Of 120 staff surveyed, 14 per cent had witnessed or experienced sexual assault by Oxfam staff. Seventy-four per cent (only four people in total, but still the majority) of staff in South Sudan had witnessed or experienced rape or attempted rape by an Oxfam staff member. Sex for aid, sex for food, and sexual abuse were common across the report. Evans took this concern to both Oxfam and the Charities Commission. She asked for additional re-sources from Oxfam to deal with the scale of concerns she was seeing. She requested follow-up meetings to discuss her reports with senior leadership but they were cancelled. The general impression was that senior leaders agreed there was an issue, but it was in hand or had been dealt with, and that measures in place were appropriate.

The Charities Commission began 'engaging' with Oxfam in 2017 about safeguarding and public allegations, before *The Times* story was published. They had agreed an action plan to be put in place in 2018, but 'events were overtaken' by story.[11] 'Engagement' became an inquiry, launched on 12 February 2018.

The Oxfam inquiry and report matters for what happened with the WHO in the DRC. Most obviously, you would assume that during a time when a major investigation into sexual abuse and exploitation was going on, other inter-national organisations working with vulnerable people in emergency contexts would check they had their house in order. Not so. There are similar patterns between what happened with Oxfam in Haiti and with the WHO in the DRC – a stressful environment, high turnover of staff, things like safeguarding falling by the wayside during an emergency, differential treatment of staff – that create conditions in which abuse and exploitation can take place. Regulation and codes of conduct can fall to the discretion of local country and regional offices. Rather than protecting the victims of abuse, there is a desire to protect the institution – Oxfam and the WHO – and the funding it receives. As the Charities Commission report notes, 'The impression the Inquiry has is that Oxfam GB's handling of these matters was influenced by a desire to protect Oxfam GB's reputation and to protect donor and stakeholder relationships.'[12] In both cases, irre-spective of proof that minors were involved, the fact that there is even an allegation involving minors suggests the issue should be addressed with urgency: this failing of Oxfam was similar to the failing of the WHO.

There is one big difference between the Oxfam and WHO cases: accountability. The *Times* headline, taken from a direct quote, was, 'It was like a Caligula orgy with prostitutes in Oxfam T-shirts',[13] and allegations of prostitution rings organised by Oxfam staff caused understandable shock and disgust among the public and politicians. The CEO of Oxfam, Mark Goldring, resigned later in the year, telling the *Guardian* he had 'faced the test of a lifetime'.[14] Having previously received £31.7 million in taxpayer money in 2016/17, Oxfam agreed to withdraw from future funding rounds from the UK government, a substantial loss to the charity's income. According to a report from the *Guardian*, a thousand direct debits were immediately cancelled and high-profile Oxfam ambassadors, from the actor Minnie Driver to the human-rights advocate Desmond Tutu, publicly resigned.[15]

In contrast, as of 2023, no member of the WHO's senior leadership team, executive board or director-general had resigned or been sacked over the DRC scandal. No senior staff member of the WHO lost their job over the rape of thirteen-year-old Jolianne. The WHO did not see a hit to their finances. Financing for the WHO predominantly comes from member countries and private philanthropy, with the top donors being the US, the UK, the EU and the Bill & Melinda Gates Foundation. Some member countries asked questions and were happy to leave it at that, others were satisfied that the WHO had launched an investigation and published the report. The overarching sense was this was all coming out at the height of the biggest health crisis of a generation – the COVID-19 pandemic – and was an unhelpful distraction: the WHO had dealt with it, so time to move on. Member states of the WHO backed the senior leadership and their claims that they did not know what was happening in the DRC at the time the abuse and exploitation took place.

In a photograph taken for the WHO during the Ebola crisis in the DRC, three men in dark navy-blue WHO flak jackets stand in elbow-bump formation. At the centre is the WHO's director-general, Tedros, smiling in sunglasses. To the right of him in the picture, wearing a black baseball cap, is the organisation's Emergency Response Team leader Michel Yao, and to the left is Boubacar Diallo. Diallo is one of the most high-profile people named in Associated Press journalists Maria Cheng and Al-Hadji Kudra Maliro's investigations into sexual abuse and exploitation in the DRC. According to their reports, Diallo offered jobs and promotions to young women working in the Ebola response in exchange for sex. He would often boast about his close relationship with Tedros.[16] Diallo has denied wrongdoing, and boasting and photographs do not mean Tedros knew about the allegations against him. But they do suggest a close enough relationship for the victims of the abuse to doubt whether they would be believed or that senior WHO management would take their side. The perpetrator deliberately used his position of power to silence the women he abused.

Tedros has stuck to his story that he did not know what was happening in the DRC until the press reports in 2020. It is a story he repeated on record to the investigation into sexual exploitation and abuse by the Independent Commission. The Associated Press investigations have consistently argued to the contrary, suggesting senior leaders including Tedros were made aware of some of the allegations as early as 2019.[17]

In February 2023, a strictly confidential report by the UN's Office of Internal Oversight Services (OIOS) was widely leaked to journalists investigating this story. While names are covered by black rectangles, you can see why staff members may have leaked the report as titles such as 'director-general' were not covered. If the leaked report is to be believed (and journalists have verified this), then it is clear that Tedros and senior management knew what was going on in the DRC in 2019. They were emailed. I doubt Tedros checks his email himself, because as director-general of the biggest health organisation in the world, he gets thousands of emails a day. But someone must have read them. Someone should have told him. He should have listened to the open secret. When there was no reply to the emails, people kept trying to raise the alarm, and these emails were followed up. Staffers in the DRC working for the WHO knew there was a major problem and tried to do the right thing by both warning the leaders and asking for help as to how to stop it, then again, and again. In the case of Diallo, three Ebola experts working in the DRC at the time informed WHO senior management and were told to leave it.[18]

When the OIOS report was published, Tedros suggested that there was confusion between the OIOS investigation and that of the Independent Commission over the legal loophole of whether a person could be defined as a victim of sexual exploitation and abuse if they were not a direct beneficiary of WHO's help. This was the loophole that the WHO itself had used to let perpetrators off the hook. Tedros claimed he wanted clarity. Sensing bullshit and deflection, the chairs of the Independent Commission took the unprecedented move of calling out the WHO (and I really can't reiterate enough how unprecedented this was: people working in the UN and international system rarely call each other out, and definitely don't do it in public), clearly stating in a press release: 'We hope that WHO will put an end to the distraction of this inappropriate academic debate over the definition of "beneficiary" and instead focus on demonstrating that its accountability system for SEA allegations is truly credible and effective.'[19]

Violence, abuse, harassment and exploitation matter and

are of serious concern, regardless of whether the victim is a colleague or a beneficiary. The beneficiary issue is a moot point: were Oxfam and the WHO staff members abusing the people they were also helping? It creates a hierarchy of harm and suggests that harm is worse if the victim is a beneficiary.

After the OIOS report was released, key member states such as the UK, the second largest donor to the WHO, came out in support of Tedros, and the 'hard work of all at WHO driving progress on PRSEAH [preventing and responding to sexual exploitation, abuse and harassment]'.[20] Against mounting evidence, senior leadership held firm that they had known nothing. Women like Jolianne were being thrown under the bus to protect the WHO and its leaders. They were being exploited all over again.

At the World Health Summit in Berlin in October 2022, a WHO senior official was accused of groping a woman. More stories emerged as to how this groper had a history of harassment that had been ignored by the organisation. Advocacy groups such as Women in Global Health started to collect stories under #healthtoo.[21] The whisper networks that had long protected women working in the WHO were going loud, and they were being heard. Journalists were on alert for stories, following up with their contacts in the DRC to search for anyone who would go on record to confront some of the worst perpetrators in the institution. On 8 February 2023, the *Telegraph* published an article about another perpetrator from the health security team in the institution's Geneva headquarters.[22] Once again there had been the warning signs, a lack of action and a perceived delay in investigating reports. But this time, the exploitation, harassment and abuse was happening to women with a profile, in the global north.

Two days after the article in the *Telegraph*, the WHO hastily pulled three senior women into its bi-weekly press briefing.

These three women – Gaya Gamhewage, who was leading the WHO's prevention and response to sexual exploitation, abuse and harassment (PRSEAH); chef de cabinet (chief operating officer) of the WHO, Catharina Boehme; and Lisa McLennon, head of investigations, OIOS – were there to show that, contrary to press reports, the WHO was trying to get a handle on things. Gamhewage had been appointed as the WHO's new head of PRSEAH. The organisation had created a dashboard recording new cases and their outcomes (e.g. dismissal, termination), and had finally got through the backlog of old cases that had been sitting in the system for ever. By early 2023, the WHO had 340 staff members as key points of contact on the matter of PRSEAH in 127 countries, including 40 staff members working full time on this issue. There was an institutional commitment to complete investigations in 120 days. For cases where perpetrators broke the law, the WHO has a survivor assistance fund, where the organisation will pay for legal aid in a country for any survivor. In 2022, after the WHO got serious, there were 107 complaints and 73 investigations, with 3 dismissals (one of which had already left the institution). The WHO does not name names for legal reasons. But it does identify the level of seniority of the perpetrators. Of the three male members of staff who had been dismissed by February 2023, one was of the highest-ranking director level – a D1 – and the other two were mid-career at P4 and P5. All of the survivors were more junior than them, with the D1 sexually harassing a female intern. Gone was the old policy that had the biggest of all loopholes – that sexual exploitation and abuse only counts as a problem if the victim is a direct beneficiary of WHO assistance – but a new policy was on its way.

The first news report on what was happening in the DRC came out in 2020, and the first formal investigation was completed in 2021. The WHO only accelerated its work on the issue once stories about attacks on women in the global north had started to accumulate in 2022/23. Black women and girls like Jolianne in the global south mattered less than white women in the global north.

The problem with the WHO stems from the culture of so many institutions that fail to put adequate systems in place to prevent and detect any acts of sexual abuse, harassment and exploitation and then follow the appropriate measures. What happened in the DRC is not a rare case of health workers in extreme countries with protracted histories of sexual violence. It happens across the WHO, from the headquarters to emergency responses. It is a problem across the global health and aid sector. Following accusations of mishandling reports of sexual abuse and harassment in the UN's HIV/AIDS organisation – UNAIDS – in 2018, the then director-general, Michel Sidibé, stepped down six months early from his leadership role.[23] He took accountability.

Tedros never took the same accountability. Member states of the WHO supported him as the person to lead the changes for the very issues he turned a blind eye to and the institutional culture he created. And when I say member states supported him, this support comes from you and your tax money. Your elected officials and the diplomats who represent your country's interests thought everything that happened in this chapter was fine, and that despite all the evidence to the contrary, WHO had got a handle on sexual abuse, exploitation and harassment, and that Tedros was the man to oversee this. For many world leaders, replacing the director-general in the middle of the COVID-19 pandemic was a step they would not take. The operations of the WHO and wider health concerns had to come first; they were the priority and the survivors of sexual abuse and exploitation a secondary concern. As Paula Donovan, head of the Code Blue Campaign to end sexual exploitation and abuse within the UN, notes, these women and girls were treated as collateral damage, something that just happens during a major health emergency.[23] It was the organisation and its male leaders who were to be protected, not the survivors of abuse and exploitation. Health first, women second. As the next chapter shows, this not only happens to women and girls subject to sexual violence by health workers, but also to women who are themselves health workers at their workplaces.

7

Attacking Health Workers, Normalising Violence Against Women

Hope always dreads the Valentine's Day shift. Most of her colleagues dread Christmas and New Year when London hospitals fill up with the excess of consumption and violence within families, and those who find a way of being admitted to hospital so they don't have to be alone over the holiday season. Not Hope – she always has a terrible shift on Valentine's Day. The first and only time she fainted at work was Valentine's Day. Then there was the year one of the patients on the ward had a cardiac arrest. But really it all came back to what happened the Valentine's Day she was a junior nurse, six months out of training.

Hope was working on her regular ward that Valentine's Day and noticed that a patient's cannula had come loose. Another routine minor problem on a routine ward. Hope quickly spotted the problem. She followed her training: reassured the patient, popped a bandage on their arm and told them she was just going to get another cannula.

BAM! 'I'M GOING TO FUCKING KILL YOU! YOU'RE

TRYING TO KILL ME! I'M GOING TO FUCKING
KILL YOU!'

Hope was forced against the wall by the patient's forearm,
which was bleeding hepatitis C-infected blood. The patient
was screaming in her face. She couldn't move. She was pinned
to the spot with the spit of death threats landing on her face.
Worried about the blood from the arm, she scanned the cor-
ridor for help.

'If you don't put her down I'm going to call security!'
shouted the senior sister on the critical care ward.

The patient put Hope down and stormed off back to
his bed.

Security were not called. The senior sister explained there
is a charge every time you call them. People were constantly
worried about budgets and overspend, so a call-out of this
kind was not worth the cost. Shaken but only six months out
of her training, Hope didn't know she could go above the
senior sister and insist security were called. She was scared
and did not want to go back and put the new cannula in the
patient's arm. Hope asked to swap patients. Her senior sister
refused. No one else wanted to care for him as he was violent:
look at what he'd just done. No thanks.

Hope did not return for her shift the next day. She said she
would only go back once he had gone or someone else was
caring for him. She waited until he had been moved on and
then carried on going to work as normal. She didn't raise what
had happened with anyone until her appraisal three months
later. Her appraisers were shocked at what had happened, not
so much by the incident as the fact that security had not been
called and this had not been reported. According to the Royal
College of Nursing, the main representative body of nurses in
the UK, employers have a legal duty to ensure places of work
are safe. Not only that, when an incident of violence occurs
it should be investigated with a review of risk-assessment

measures.[1] You can imagine how popular a review of risk-assessment measures would be with an overworked senior sister who most likely knows they need more help but none is forthcoming. As the newest nurse on the ward, Hope should have been supported better by her line manager, but her line manager should also be better supported by her employer.

Hope is now a senior nurse working in critical care. The Valentine's Day incident sticks in her head but it's definitely not the only case of violence she has seen. She has seen patients 'smash up the place' and one colleague seriously injured when their head was battered against a wall. As Hope told me, 'there's always one' at any given time. Working in critical care nursing like she is now, you come to expect violence as patients can respond in different ways when emerging from heavy sedation. Because of this, senior nurses try to ensure there is a trained mental health nurse on shift to help deal with patients when they come around. However, as Hope explained to me, these shifts are 'impossible to fill'. Mental health nurses are overstretched and find critical care work challenging. She copes as best she can. Or, as she put it to me, she copes by 'being a sexist' and making the male nurses on shift deal with the violent cases. The male nurses (understandably) complain that they always have the difficult patients and there is not always a male nurse on duty, but Hope is pretty pragmatic: she is not going to deal with a 'big scary man' again.

Nurses are subjected to more violence than any other type of health worker, to the extent that in the UK such violence is routinely recognised as 'a significant occupational hazard for nursing and midwifery staff'.[2] Hope is just one of the one in four UK nurses who have experienced verbal or physical violence in their workplace. The odds are worse for nurses and midwifes with 'protected characteristics',[3] i.e. nurses and midwives of colour, with disabilities, or transgender health workers.

The official data we have on how many health workers experience violence around the world is shockingly poor. The WHO puts the global number of incidents of violence at between 8 and 38 per cent of health workers – a vague and highly imprecise statistic that doesn't tell us much.[4] Leading authorities in the health sector around the world agree that both the violence and lack of data on it is a prevalent problem. The joint taskforce on workplace violence in the health sector – an alliance between the WHO, International Labour Organization (ILO), International Council of Nurses and Public Services International – asserted that such violence is a structural issue, i.e. embedded in the culture and working practices of health, way back in 2002.[5] Yet, we still don't have good global data on the scale of the structural issue. Just this weird 8 to 38 per cent statistic and the odd anecdote from small, national-based surveys. Violence against health workers is normalised as something that just happens.

This is particularly relevant to women because women make up 70 per cent of health workers in the world. Women are not only the majority of health workers, they are over-represented in front-line work, from A&E receptionists to nurses to community care teams. It is front-line health workers – particularly those working in acute care, mental health and ambulance services – who are more likely to be subjected to violence from patients and their families. Hence, violence against health workers is a form of violence against women: as I unpack below, it shows a lack of respect for the roles women occupy, and it is neglected because it is seen as a normal, everyday occupational hazard in women's working lives.

When I asked Hope how management responded to her concerns when she raised it in her appraisal, she shrugged off my question, because it is just accepted as one of those things, part of the job. The NHS in England has attempted to do something about violence against nurses such as Hope, publishing a Violence Prevention and Reduction Standard in 2020 outlining its approach to the issue. But workers like the senior sister who didn't call security have so many competing demands on their time and budget because of day to day firefighting that there is little incentive to implement such an approach, despite the clear benefits for their staff. Moreover, the extent of physical and verbal threats and acts of violence have become so normalised that many health workers, like Hope, shrug it off. There is the practical shrug: if working in a high-pressured environment such as an emergency room or critical care unit in a busy hospital, you just do the de-escalation training in how to handle the risk of violence and get on with your job. You know, as one study for the NHS confirmed, that de-escalation training won't reduce the number of incidents of violence.[6] One nurse pointed out to me that what they really need instead of de-escalation training is escalation training: showing nurses how they can escalate issues to their bosses to make them take action. Worrying about it won't stop it happening: better to be prepared and then move on. There is also the more macho shrug: if you can't handle this aspect of medicine, do something else, as if being subjected to high-pressure tension and violence is a badge of honour.

Shrugging it off individualises the problem. Either you take practical steps to deal with the issue (take self-defence classes, work on your mediation skills or get a friend to screenshot, block and report if online abuse) or you toughen up. The solution is up to individuals like Hope, not her employer, and definitely not the government or wider health system. Nurses around the world are developing individual ways to reduce the threat of violence – buddying up for clinic consultations, beeping each other at intervals to check in, moving their desks away from patients and nearer to the exit, making sure only one person is on the phone at any time so another can jump on the line and caution a family member if they are threatening their colleague. None of this solves the problem. It's akin to the measures you take when you come back from a night out with your friends – call me when you get in, I'll track your cab, hold your keys in your hand. We think these measures make us safer, but they don't deal with the problem of violence against women, who commits the violence and where, and whether they are ever reported or prosecuted. Nurses, like all women, find small ways of coping and adjusting to the threat of violence, fed up with waiting for those in power to do something about it. It makes people quit the profession, or leads to a large number of health workers signed off work on account of burnout, stress, depression and/or anxiety about being attacked, or going into another area of medicine. Individualising the problem makes it worse for everyone, including under-staffed hospitals and clinics.

The US campaign group No Silence on ED Violence point out that nurses in America see the problem as 'endemic' to their workplace. In an article called 'Nothing Changes, Nobody Cares', the group recognises key cues, individual identifiers linked to patients (e.g. under the influence of drugs or alcohol) and environmental situations that, combined, make up a series of trends that can help predict – and therefore mitigate against – attacks against health workers.[7] All too often, there is no administrative support or 'judicial recourse' for such violence. In the US specifically, few cases are prosecuted, and there is a lack of understanding by both hospital administrators and law enforcement.[8] Violence could be preventable by identifying key cues and triggers. But this does not happen.

The WHO acknowledges attacks on health workers are a problem, that nurses are the worst affected, and that any approach to tackling the issue should 'attack the problem at its roots, involve all parties concerned and take into account the special cultural and gender-dimensions of the problem'.[9] The WHO then outlines its favourite go-to recommendations when it lacks knowledge and inspiration on an issue: more research, more training and greater sensitivity to cultural and gender issues. How to be culturally and gender sensitive comes down to women themselves: women need to be empowered, and in turn work practices need to make sure night workers, especially women, move between spaces together in health settings, which I take to mean don't walk around your place of work alone at night, even if you're on a night shift.[10] Another article on the issue in the *BMJ* suggests the solution is for women to find their voice and co-ordinate action on the problem, build shared understanding and make professional organisations more balanced.[11]

Like other forms of violence against women, violence against health workers is so normalised it is hiding in plain sight, there is no good data on it and somehow the onus is on women to prevent it. Women healthcare workers deserve so much more than this.

'Don't worry, love, you should see the other woman.'

I was failing not to stare at the woman sat next to me outside Manchester Royal Infirmary on the cusp of Friday night into Saturday morning. She offered me a cigarette as she tried to smoke hers while telling me about the fight she won through a mouthful of blood and missing teeth. If you've been to an emergency room in a major city on a Friday night you may recognise this scene. The low thrum of violence, the high intensity of life and death, and minor injuries just waiting to be seen. Pain and impatience are a toxic combination, and frustration builds up as people wait for hours to be put out of agony, or lash out on account of being drunk, high, scared or confused. And the people subject to this lashing out are the first people patients see – nurses, porters and receptionists.

It is in emergency healthcare that the highest number of attacks against health workers happen. According to No Silence on ED Violence, over half of emergency physicians have been assaulted in the US, with 70 per cent of emergency nurses reporting having been hit or kicked by patients.[12] Violence can be physical or verbal, including threats of future harm. For example, according to a survey by the American College of Emergency Physicians, 83 per cent of emergency physicians had received threats from patients saying they would return to hurt them.[13] The causes of such violence follow a clear set of trends: long waiting times, a high percentage of psychiatric patients with a history of violence, and patients under the influence of drugs and alcohol.[14]

In April 2020, a twenty-seven-year-old man in Manchester was sent to prison for two years for fracturing an NHS worker's cheekbone. He lashed out at the health worker after they'd told him they did not have any juice for him to drink, only water. The attacker was of 'no fixed address' and was in hospital following a drug overdose.[15] It does not take much to work out this man was potentially a homeless drug addict, and therefore fitted a certain risk category of someone who may become agitated or violent. He could have been flagged as a risk and proper measures taken to protect the health worker. This is the sort of incident that happens time and time again in emergency health work around the world.

A leading expert on violence against health workers, Larissa Fast, reasserted this point to me when discussing measures to prevent violence against health workers. She told me the story of a paramedic who ended up with a broken jaw, similarly to the Manchester case, from a man with a history of violence against health workers. The broken jaw could have been avoided if the perpetrator had been noted in the system:

a red flag would have been raised when he placed his call, and appropriate measures could have been taken to protect the paramedic. But there was no red flag in the system: the hospital didn't keep a record of previous incidents because of concerns about reputational damage, and not wanting to scare its staff. As Fast put it to me, 'When you do start paying attention in some ways, it is then where do you stop? It is constant violence. And then if you start collecting data on it then it ratchets up the fear level because people start becoming aware and are like, oh my god, it's so dangerous I can't do that.'

The Manchester man who broke the jaw of a health worker over a box of juice was sent to prison. The maximum sentence for assaulting a health worker in the UK was doubled from one to two years' prison time in 2020 – this is a harsher punishment than common assault which has a maximum prison time of six months in the UK (unless racially or religiously motivated, which can lead to up to two years in prison). An act of violence should be investigated and met with the appropriate punishment. However, punitive approaches alone overlook some of the root causes of aggression and how they go beyond individuals. Take long waiting times as an example. Anyone who has used any over-burdened health service knows how infuriating long waiting times can be, though hopefully have not taken that fury out on staff. Beyond simple decency, there is no point taking that fury out on staff as there is little they can do about it. Waiting times are a problem of funding and staffing shortfalls that lie squarely at the feet of national governments and how much money they are willing to invest in their health service and wider social care provision. Take another example: patients with poor mental health and/or drug dependencies. Again, there is very little health practitioners can do for them without the proper resourcing for health, social security, welfare and addiction support, especially for the most marginalised and poor in society. This is why some senior leaders working within the NHS are cautious about 'zero-tolerance' approaches to violence against healthcare workers. They think that zero tolerance would end up punishing the most marginalised in society, and what is needed is a more wholesale reform of the culture of the NHS.[16]

Politicians only care about violence against health workers when it suits them. 'Zero tolerance' towards the issue has been in the headlines three times in the UK: once when Tony Blair's government introduced the 1999 Health Act, when taking prominent action on violence was a way of showing commitment to health workers during a time of increased privatisation. In 2005, during the general election campaign, spokespeople for all major parties promised action on attacks on health workers. Most recently, during COVID-19, when the public's love of health workers was at an all-time high and trust in the government at a major low, the policy resurfaced. But even then, this love did not last long, with the NHS's violence prevention and reduction (VPR) team expressing concern to the *Guardian* in 2023 that their team was about to be cut and all the work carried out by the NHS and police deprioritised.[17] Governments only care about health and care workers when they need to be seen to be caring. Outside an emergency, policy launch or election cycle, such violence is normalised and little is being done to address it.

In the first six months of the COVID-19 pandemic, the International Committee of the Red Cross (ICRC) reported 611 known incidents of attacks on health workers in non-conflict settings.[18] The number was likely to have been much higher as such violence is so under-reported, especially during a major pandemic. India and Mexico had two of the highest numbers of attacks during the first two years of COVID-19.[19] India was already 'one of the most unsafe countries for health workers', with health workers being four times more likely to be assaulted than any other professional.[20] In Mexico, high numbers of health workers were subject to violence out of fear that they were spreading the virus. Workers were targeted in their homes, in public spaces such as restaurants, and online.[21] GP surgeries in the UK saw 'unprecedented abuse' from patients, and in 2020 England saw a 30 per cent increase of abuse against ambulance staff.[22] The *Nursing Times* reported nurses being spat at and called 'disease spreaders',[23] which would be a comic irony if it were not so disgusting. Across the world, from the Philippines to Myanmar, health workers who were once proud to walk their neighbourhoods in their uniforms started to change out of their clothes, fearing being attacked by their community. At a point in world history where you would assume health workers would be valued and rewarded, the risk of violence against them went up, not down.

The rise in public awareness of attacks on health workers during COVID-19 led to some further government action in some countries. In India, for example, the government passed an emergency amendment to the Emergency Epidemic Laws so such attacks could lead to up to seven years in prison. Prominent scientific advisers such as US Chief Medical Advisor Anthony Fauci were assigned personal security or, in the case of Belgian virologist Marc Van Ranst, moved to a safe house.[24] Most measures were reactionary, piecemeal and failed to tackle other forms of violence such as online abuse where health experts – and in some cases their families – were subject to threats of violence and death, intimidation, offensive comments and abusive challenges to their expertise in response to something they'd said in the media, on vaccines, or the latest government initiative. No measure to protect health workers and experts during COVID-19 was specific to the needs of women. While prominent male leaders got increased protection, there was less attention directed towards protecting front-line health workers, and hence the women that make up the majority of these positions. No one was protecting women in their place of work, and no one was protecting them online. They were on their own.

As soon as the COVID-19 vaccines started to roll out across the UK, senior midwives started to worry. Research showed that 98 per cent of pregnant women who were admitted to hospital with COVID-19 between May and July 2021 had not been vaccinated, and of those in hospital, one-third had to receive respiratory support, over a third developed pneumonia and one in seven needed intensive care. The worry was twofold. First, that the message that COVID-19 vaccines were safe for pregnant women was not getting out. And second, that pregnant women were not aware of the risks of not being vaccinated. Evidence suggested that pregnant women with COVID-19 symptoms at the time of birth would be more likely to need a C-section, develop pre-eclampsia, and have higher risk of premature and still birth.

The three main leaders of maternity healthcare issued clear statements encouraging women to get vaccinated. One of them, the chief midwifery officer for England, Jacqueline Dunkley-Bent, stated the safety of the vaccines, the risks to mother and baby of not getting vaccinated and the need for 'everyone to come forward and take up the evergreen offer of a jab which is why I am calling on pregnant women to take action to protect themselves and their babies and on my fellow midwives to ensure they have the information they need to do so.'[25] In response to her 'It is safer to be vaccinated' tweet, @Pedro91662106 replied: 'Looking forward to Nuremberg 2?'[26]

This painting of Professor Dunkley-Bent as a Nazi was mere everyday abuse compared to the Nazi-Bitch-Die-Scum-Evil-Mother-Child-Killer torrent against her colleague Gill Walton, chief executive and general secretary of the Royal College of Midwives. Walton was called an 'evil bitch' and compared to the child murderer Myra Hindley.[27] All Walton had done was issue a clear statement based on evidence from the research she had seen, in support of the official guidance for pregnant women.[28]

Far from staying silent in the face of abuse against one of their own, the health community rallied around Gill Walton. The Royal College of Midwives retweeted the abuse and reported it to Twitter/X, and colleagues expressed online solidarity with #IstandwithGill. What was concerning about the abuse was it was not an isolated incident. The Royal College of Midwives had seen an upswing in abuse against midwives, specifically around vaccines.[29]

A study by the medical journal *Nature* of 321 scientists who offered public commentary on COVID-19 suggested two topics triggered the most online abuse: vaccines and the origins of COVID-19. Abuse varied from the usual threats of violence and death to attacks on experts' credibility. For example, one Australian female virologist, who sought to defend the professionalism of colleagues working in Wuhan, was sent an email with the subject line: 'Eat a bat and die, bitch.'[30] While the study did not identify any specific trends as to the gendered nature of abuse, one expert who had been subject to abuse in the study noted, 'If you're a woman, or a person of colour from a marginalised group, that abuse will probably include your personal characteristics.'[31]

Online abuse, particularly against women, is an accepted way of life on social media. As the feminist campaigner Laura Bates argues in her book *Men Who Hate Women*, online misogyny spills over into in schools, universities, government, the workplace and every aspect of society, including hospitals, doctor's surgeries and labour wards.[32] Online abuse targets health workers directly at their work through threatening emails, in addition to other forms of communication such as abusive phone calls. These are often from the family of patients.

The UK has a serious midwife shortage. As of 2020, one in five midwife positions were unfulfilled.[33] Shortages create increased burdens on the existing workforce, which can increase stress. Add some in-person and online abuse and you can see why this staffing problem may persist and worsen. Abuse against healthcare workers is not only a problem for the mental and physical well-being and safety of the majority of women who make up this specialised workforce. It will also have knock-on effects for the health, safety and well-being of women and pregnant people and their babies.

Violence is a normalised part of working in the health sector and it shouldn't be. While all health workers at every level are subject to violence, it is the front-line positions – the positions predominantly staffed by women – that are the most vulnerable. The solutions we have to these problems often acknowledge it is front-line health workers and nurses bearing the brunt. But we so rarely hear about gender. Violence of this kind is either normalised or not recognised precisely because of who is vulnerable: women.

To take this issue seriously, violence against health workers needs to be seen for what it is: gender-based violence. It is a form of gender-based violence: women are more susceptible to this violence because the health work they do – care work, nursing – is devalued as women's work, meaning governments don't act on the problem. When you devalue women and their work, you devalue their need to be safe. Devaluing a role grants a licence to someone to be abusive or violent. The woman in front of them is 'just' a nurse or a paramedic, is 'just' doing the immediate care; they're not the doctors or surgeons who do the real work. Same goes for 'just' the receptionist, cleaner or hospital social worker. If you don't value these roles, you don't value the person doing them, and accept that any harm that comes to them is 'just' part of the job. Healthcare work being women's work means violence is tolerated and not acted upon, and under-reported and under-researched. Risk and inaction around violence against health work is gendered: there is not enough data on it, like so many issues that affect women, and not enough provision to stop it from happening because it happens to women.

Violence against women workers in health settings – be it abuse, injury or calling someone a child murderer on social media – is the most everyday form of women as collateral within failing health systems. The most acute forms of abuse do not just happen in extreme situations such as war zones, but in the heart of the community and on our social media feeds. This not only has a huge impact on the health and well-being of health workers themselves, but on the patients and communities they serve as more workers leave the profession or shift away from critical and emergency care roles. Gender-based violence against health workers should concern us as a form of violence against women, and as a major driver of under-staffing of health systems. As the next chapter shows, it is no wonder so many health workers are at risk of burnout, and are wanting to leave the profession.

8

Burnt out and Quitting

She receives the first phone call from a panicked doctor at 8.30 a.m. He is shouting at her to come quickly. This is before she has turned on her laptop or looked at her list of patients to see. She attends to the stressed doctor and goes back to her desk. The phone rings again. The pattern repeats itself. After a moment of peace, she is off to morning clinic. She reviews patient diagnoses, treatment and care plans. Crucially, she has to assess how quickly she can get them home. She will see on average five patients in a morning, spending forty-five minutes with each where she can, longer if they have a difficult care or home situation, or if the patient or their family are frightened. She thinks it's her job to take time. So she tries. Then a doctor will ask her to squeeze in another patient. But it is her who is being endlessly squeezed. A doctor shouts at her again. Why has this patient not been moved on? The countdown on her laptop is ticking. She needs to refer the patient admitted at 3 a.m. She has to get patients moved: onto the ward, out of the hospital. She starts to process patient exits, travel plans, home medical and care plans, financial plans. She gets another call. The emergency department. Another suicide case. She leaves her paperwork and gets to emergency.

The clock ticks. She will need to process the care plan. She has two hours to move the patient at risk of suicide, twenty-two hours less than a normal patient. She is meant to leave at 5.55 p.m. but she will stay until 7 p.m. She has to leave then to preserve herself. She knows she is the one who leaves first. Others stay until 9 p.m. The phone rings again. This time it's the palliative care team. She is needed for a family conference. Family conferences take time. She is straight off to the intensive care unit. She returns to her desk and realises she hasn't eaten. She can't do this any more. She has to leave. She is the most senior medical social worker in the hospital. She is needed. In 2019 she quit.

Rai loved her job. As a medical social worker specialising in renal medicine, she takes pride in her work. She sees herself as an invaluable part of the health system, someone who connects patients, families, social care and the medical teams. She is the lynchpin in hospitals like the ones she worked in in Singapore and Hong Kong. Without her, the patients can't move on. She is fundamental to assessing their care packages and what they need inside and outside the hospital environment. This is why she is one of the key members of the on-call rota for the emergency room. Any signs of suicide, family violence or elder abuse and the emergency room staff call Rai.

In the end she left her job because she couldn't take the constant calls for her help, the pressure to move patients on, the shouting from doctors, the clock ticking down to deadline. She was used to it but something had started to shift. People came to work looking like they had been crying. She saw the physical and emotional pain in her colleagues. Not only did she have to process the emotional impact of her work, but the culture of her line management started to change. There was less time to learn about patients. Management knew society was getting older and there was a crisis in getting enough people to care for the ageing population. But no one wanted to create a budget for this. It was falling on people like her, the medical social workers caught between an ageing population, cuts in care roles, changing demography so that less care of the elderly was happening in the home, and full hospitals with older patients with nowhere to go and no one to care for them. As Rai explained to me, care for the ageing population was the one thing you 'can't rely on the robots' for.

Rai tried talking to her manager. They told her just to handle it. This is the job. Then they gave her a junior colleague to manage. Line management and training added to her workload. She wanted to protect the junior colleague from the worst of the stress. She told her manager she planned to quit. They referred her to CBT (cognitive behavioural therapy). It didn't work. Planning her day and doing something nice didn't cut it when she had patients who needed her or colleagues taking out their stress on her. Another colleague referred her to art therapy. Art therapy was great. It helped her express herself. She expressed to her manager that she was quitting.

According to a global survey of health workers, Hong Kong tops the table for health-worker burnout. Forty-six per cent of workers said they worked over fifty hours a week, and 61 per cent felt unwell because of their work-related stress.[1] Like it was for Rai, the cause of this burnout is a toxic combination of long work hours, lack of physical and mental space, poor job security and career opportunities, bullying and a culture of stress. All of which is compounded by an ageing population with increased healthcare needs. Hong Kong has always had a high turnover of health workers. However, this notably increased in 2021 on account of the COVID-19 pandemic and an emigration wave. Health workers were quitting, leaving or emigrating. This may have been good for the workers who left, but it was terrible for those who stayed.

Rai now lives and works in China. She is still a senior medical social worker but she is freelance and sets her own hours. While the job is stressful, she can manage the stress on her own terms. She worked during the COVID-19 pandemic, remotely supporting colleagues working in Wuhan in the early stages of the outbreak. With COVID-19 she felt she was needed and that she was appreciated. When we spoke, she told me that the most important part of her experience with burnout is that she can now see it in others. She is sensitive to the signs. She can try and stop it from getting as bad as it was for her. She doesn't want anyone else to go through the despair that she did.

Rai's story may seem extreme, but it is a common one. Burnout affects all genders. And gender norms – such as the expectation that men need to be strong and confident in the workplace and not talk about their feelings; or dealing with constant use of the wrong pronouns and lack of recognition, and therefore respect, if you're non-binary or trans; or the assumption you'll take on more tasks out of love and care if you're a woman – all work in different ways to influence how people experience and manage burnout. Why these gendered norms affect women more than men is again because of the sheer number of women in the health workforce and how the phenomenon of burnout concentrates around feminised labour. Hong Kong follows a similar pattern to the rest of the world, with a feminised workforce, especially at the front line. According to a 2017 government assessment of staff, while 68 per cent of doctors in Hong Kong are male, 100 per cent of midwives, 85 per cent of nurses, 67 per cent of occupational therapists and 54 per cent of lab technicians and physiotherapists are female.[2] The majority of workers burnt out by the Hong Kong health system are women like Rai.

In 2019, the WHO classified burnout as a syndrome in the International Classification of Diseases. This was the first time burnout had a formal classification, an important step for many occupational health advocates who had been wanting greater recognition and clarity around the term. According to the WHO definition, 'Burnout is a syndrome conceptualized as resulting from chronic workplace stress that has not been successfully managed.'[3]

There are three elements to this definition: 1. 'feeling of energy depletion or exhaustion'; 2. 'increased mental distance from one's job or feelings of negativism or cynicism related to one's job'; and 3. 'reduced professional efficacy'. What is fundamental to the definition is that burnout is an *occupational* health issue. It's all about work demands, poor management and increased stress. You can't get burnout from other aspects of your life. If you're feeling burnt out from the monotony of endless ironing and washing, packed lunches, diary planning, neighbourhood/school/nursery group messages, shopping, cooking, cleaning, moving children around from school to sports to playdates, and even more washing, with no thanks or progression, all while everyone around you assumes all you do is watch daytime TV while doomscrolling, then – sorry – you cannot be burnt out. Someone has to have mismanaged you and your stress. Burnout therefore excludes a huge swathe of labour that women do. You can be tired of being a full-time carer for your family or wider community, exhausted even, but it is not the same as burnout.

Burnout may not be formally recognised in some aspects of women's labour, but it is acute in other areas. Burnout is more likely in jobs such as teaching and healthcare work: women's work.[4] Some studies estimate that a third of all health workers have experienced burnout during their careers.[5] And that this is 'more burdensome for front-line junior physicians' and primary health workers.[6] As far back as 1996, the ILO published guidelines on work-related stress in nursing (which were still the main guidelines the ILO were using in 2022), noting, 'Nursing is acknowledged to be stressful work, and there is a need to understand the nature of that problem and to better manage it.'[7]

Given what we've seen in the other chapters – abuse, assault and violence – it is no wonder that many working in the health sector experience burnout. These are clearly unsafe working conditions. However, it is not just these extreme issues facing the health workforce around the world. It is also the minutiae of everyday poor management. It is constantly having to measure and record your performance against KPIs (key performance indicators) and the resulting reduced time you have to engage with patients and your colleagues. Continuous reform and changes to the health sector can result in constant restructuring, administrative burden and frustration that once again health reform is being used as a political tool. It is about putting your patients first at the cost of your own well-being, as you worry that if you don't no one else will.

Health workers of colour have to contend with these pressures and the added stress of racist harassment, bullying and discrimination. Such harassment, bullying and discrimination can happen in spaces where they are the minority or majority ethnic group. Health systems and facilities often reflect wider inequalities in society. Racism is a structural problem in society: even where workers of colour make up the majority in a health setting they can still face racism. In systems with severe racism and racial inequality, be it in one country or the overall international aid system, health workers of colour are going to be more burdened by the stress of micro and macro racism.

Burnout is a cyclical problem. Under-staffing, early retirement and colleagues leaving because of burnout all put increased pressure on workers. This pressure leads them to burn out and leave the profession temporarily or for good. This doubles down on the pressure and the cycle continues. The dangerous point is when burnout becomes the norm and staff recruitment cannot keep up with the numbers of people leaving the profession. This is the burnout double whammy: it affects individuals, but if not addressed it also becomes a systemic problem that spreads throughout the sector.

Like many of the issues discussed in this book, the people in charge of health systems around the world know burnout is a problem and are increasingly worried about it. This is less because of the impact it is having on individual staff and more because it causes chaos in their health systems. For health managers, the biggest problem is patients: you don't want burnt-out health professionals treating patients, because this often has deadly, costly and political consequences.

According to the World Health Assembly resolution on 'protecting, safeguarding, and investing in the health and care workforce':

> the physical and mental health and well-being of health and care workers is impacted by health-worker and skills shortages that can contribute to increased stress, workload, and burnout; and decreased health-worker productivity, performance and retention – resulting in enduring effects on the functioning, efficiency and resiliency of health systems; and concerned that the world, if the current trends continue, *could suffer from a projected shortfall of 18 million health workers in 2030, primarily in low- and lower-middle-income countries.*[8]

In addition, 400 million people will lack basic access to healthcare.[9] The pain of these shortfalls will mostly be felt by people living in low- and middle-income countries in Africa, Latin America and South East Asia. However, the trend is global. In the UK, the Nursing and Midwifery Council reported 27,000 nurses and midwives left the official register in 2020, a 13 per cent rise from the previous year, with a third reporting pressure and workplace stress as their reason for doing so.[10] This is undoubtedly linked to the extreme working conditions during COVID-19, but concerns about health-worker shortages pre-date the pandemic and only go some way to explain the wider potential 18 million-person shortfall in health workers in the world. As the WHO suggests, the health workforce is the backbone of any health system.

The proposed solutions to these problems are a mix of calls to action from international bodies telling governments what they should be doing (which they often ignore) and guidance for health managers. Management guidance tends to focus on the obvious: clear and consistent goal-setting, training, mentoring, 'culturally appropriate' staff support, support groups, buy-in on decision-making, identifying the cause of stress, risk assessments and more training on 'conflict resolution'.[11] On the world stage there is no end of acknowledgments, recognitions, reaffirmations and resolutions (to use the language of the UN) in committing to health-worker well-being. There is general agreement that something must be done! There are initiatives, technical guidance and codes of practice. But not so many people are willing to do what must be done.

It is all well and good for politicians and health leaders to say they care about something, but to see if something is being taken seriously you need to look at the boring stuff: strategy, action plans, targets and indicators. With burnout, some governments have reports, commissions and/or inquiries on the issue, but rarely strategies. The Health and Social Care Committee of the UK's House of Commons, for example, published a sixty-six-page report on burnout in the NHS and social care system, and flagged the need for the health and social care system to do more and be better. In a damning conclusion, the report noted that burnout was so great it would require a 'total overhaul':

The emergency that workforce burnout has become will not be solved without a total overhaul of the way the NHS does workforce planning. ... The way that the NHS does workforce planning is at best opaque and at worst responsible for the unacceptable pressure on the current workforce which existed even before the pandemic.[12]

However, if you look at the plan for this potential 'overhaul' in the document, 'We are the NHS: People Plan 2020/21 – action for us all', it is quite meek. Burnout is acknowledged in the fifty-two-page plan, but only in an explanatory box on 'Support to switch off from work'.[13] The recognition and recommendations for change are rarely met with the will or strategies to do so. The burden is on the burnt-out worker to sort it out for themselves.

On the global stage, there are no real action plans. Take, for example, the WHO's 'Workforce 2030' strategy. Given the WHO's panic about a shortage of health workers and its relationship to burnout, I thought the strategy would be full of recommendations. Not so. Burnout, stress and/or fatigue are not mentioned once. Neither are they in the WHO's Global Code of Practice on Recruitment. Instead there is a great deal of emphasis on 'optimising health worker satisfaction'[14] and building and sustaining a resilient health workforce. Same with the WHO's guideline on self-care interventions for health and well-being: there are plenty of recommendations to 'empower' individuals, communities and health workers to attend to their own health and well-being. These recommendations are presented as 'the most promising and exciting' solutions to the global crisis in healthcare provision. But there is very little on how to transform health systems to help health workers. On the contrary, it is health workers who are going to be leading this change by demonstrating good practice to 'clients'.[15] There is definitely no mention as to how this may impact on women more than men. It seems that burnout is something acknowledged by governments and health leaders but not something to be included in workforce strategies. Again, here is an issue that affects women more than men, will have huge consequences for women's professional lives and a significant impact on the quality of healthcare we receive, with potentially devastating consequences. And yet ... nothing.

It falls into the trap of just being one of those things that we all accept. Workers accept that their job may be stressful. Managers accept that the work environment is stressful and that this will lead to high turnover. Burnout is normalised as part of healthcare work in the same way violence was in the last chapter, because it impacts primarily on women and women's work.

In March 2020, the month when the UK went into its first COVID-19 lockdown, a series of pictures began to appear during my social-media doomscrolling. Doctors, nurses and anaesthetists, particularly those who had been working in ICUs (intensive care units) around the world, started posting selfies of their faces after work. These faces were shattered, solemn and covered in red blotches, bruising and imprints left by the masks and PPE they had been wearing for over ten hours. For some, this PPE had been improvised because of poor government procurement. For all, the images were to show the world what it looked and felt like working on the front line of the COVID-19 response. One post by anaesthesia registrar Natalie Silvey showed her face marked with red dents after working a nine-hour shift on 21 March 2020. It was accompanied by the comment, 'I feel broken – and we are only at the start.'[16] The tweet received 13k comments, 405.7k likes and 118.2k retweets. The comments featured pictures of other health professionals coming off shift with similar red dents, and positive messages from celebrities thanking Silvey for all she was doing. People were seeing what was happening to health workers. The posts worked: they went viral around the world, and people demanded better PPE and care for shattered health workers.

As we saw in the last chapter, COVID-19 made many things in the health sector and the lives of health workers worse. Burnout during COVID-19 was exacerbated by working conditions and practices, guidance that changed all the time, reduced staff–patient ratios, lack of standardisation, poor PPE and guilt over potentially bringing a lethal virus home to family members and loved ones.[17] It increased stress, fatigue and cynicism. It also brought attention to what health workers were facing, the impact of stress and burnout on their lives and a focus on the gender of front-line health workers. Studies, surveys and articles about the well-being and stress of doctors and nurses started to crop up in the main British and American medical journals – the *BMJ* and *JAMA*.[18] The *Lancet* published a call to action letter, noting 'this burnout has reached an alarmingly high rate', a 'tipping point' globally, and that 'this pandemic is acutely highlighting the damaging mental health consequences being faced by women in medicine'.[19] Workers sought out support, either through informal WhatsApp groups and support networks, or more formal initiatives such as the UK's *Nursing Times* 'Are you okay?' campaign, which sought to provide psychological support for nurses during the pandemic.

The risk is that during a crisis everyone is focused on the event, not those responding to it. Protect your health workers is great political rhetoric but becomes rapidly empty in practice. Their well-being becomes secondary. It is only once the fatigue and burnout starts to show that support groups are formed and initiatives start to kick in. Sadly, this is often too late for those who go on to have long-term health issues because of their work. Once the crisis passes, it is back to burnt-out business as usual. Or it is until health workers do decide to take action, by stepping away from the profession altogether, or going on strike.

It was a glorious morning as I walked over London Bridge in December 2022, all clear blue skies and buzzing tourists stopping for selfies in front of Tower Bridge. Across the bridge, tucked behind the Southbank Centre and the shadow of London's biggest phallus, the Shard, an apron of nurses stood outside Guy's and St Thomas' hospital, decked out in the navy hats of the Royal College of Nursing, with official and home-made placards. The nurses stood outside the hospital that day as part of the largest strike in the 106-year history of the Royal College of Nursing.

As I surveyed the placards along the picket line, two grabbed my attention: 'NHS HERO but my purse says zero' and 'Can't Eat, Can't Care, Claps R work thin air'. Impressed by anyone who can think of what to write on a sign other than 'Treat me better, please', I approached the women holding the placards to see why they were there. As we began to chat, the three young women with the placards explained how they had got their pins in the last two years. One had left Ireland to get better pay in the UK. This was not her first picket. The other two, from England, were new and nervous about strike action. One had arrived at the picket at 7 a.m. – she felt so emotional about the action that she had woken up early. The three young nurses absolutely knew why they were on strike – for their patients and the sense that things had to get better. People were leaving all the time, the workload was getting greater and greater, the feeling of burnout worse. The NHS needed a new word for crisis. These three talented nurses, who had only qualified two years earlier, who were full of laughter and insight when I was talking to them and who clearly cared about their patients and colleagues, were already thinking about leaving the health workforce.

As I chatted with the nurses on the picket, each told me the number-one reason they were taking industrial action was because of patients. Patient safety, patient care. The more senior nurses were also there for the junior nurses. They were concerned about their university debt, how they could afford to live in London and to pay for their commute, let alone food. One nurse told me that when she was starting out she would have to take on four extra shifts – effectively doing two weeks' work in one – if she wanted to do anything other than go to work, pay her rent, eat basic food, sleep and repeat. Holidays, going out, hobbies, presents for family and friends' birthdays were a luxury that depended on overwork.

The nurses' strike of December 2022 was only the second time that nurses in the UK had ever taken industrial action. Prior to 1995, the Royal College had banned nurses from going on strike. You can see why: nurses are the backbone of health systems, dealing with life or death. To go on strike is a huge risk. The same is true when doctors, firefighters and ambulance crews go on strike. This is partly why politicians and health leaders try to stop health workers going on strike – because of the impact it will have on people's health and the risk people may die as a consequence. But politicians and health leaders also know that most of the public will most likely side with nurses. Striking health workers and unions make every effort to let the public know that; before going on strike, they put protections in place to minimise harm, and should a major crisis happen, nurses would cross the picket to help. More importantly, most people have first-hand experience of how nurses and health and care professionals have gone above and beyond for them or someone they love. Taking industrial action is never the easy option for workers, especially nurses, and extreme action reflects their extreme work situation.

The 2022–3 nurses' strike was a part of a wider wave of industrial action of health workers in the UK. The official line is nurses went on strike in the UK in 2022 over low pay and chronic under-staffing that put patients at risk and created poor working conditions. These factors are ripe ingredients for health-worker burnout and making people want to leave the profession. Throughout 2022–3, members of the major health trade unions all voted for strike action on account of pay, working conditions and patient safety and care: ambulance crews, consultants, physiotherapists and junior doctors all withdrew their labour. It was not just health workers in the UK doing this. Between 2020 and 2023, there was national and regional industrial action by health workers in Spain, Romania, Belgium, Italy, Australia, New Zealand, Malaysia, South Korea and the US – all over the same issues. The leaders of health systems around the world had left it to health workers to deal with burnout themselves, so they did. They took action and fought back.

Picket lines are full of goodwill – delivery drivers honking their horns, strangers bringing homemade cakes, cafés offering hot drinks and the use of their loo for those striking. They are where people put their nerves aside to fight together for better working conditions, better care for patients. The picket outside the hospital in south London represented what trade-union membership and British health workers look like: predominantly women, a mix of ethnic diversity, all ages. Women make up the majority of trade-union membership, in part because union membership in the UK is heavily skewed towards the public sector, and women dominate public-sector industries such as health and education. It's also because women are taking a stand on gender pay gaps, discrimination and harassment at work through union membership. The health sector is at the forefront of this: women like the nurses on the picket wanting a change to their working conditions and our health service. Goodwill is what the NHS is built on and it is in desperately short supply. One nurse told me it had never been this bad: not only is there no goodwill any more, but people are starting to turn on each other. Pickets may be the only part of the NHS where there is any goodwill. But goodwill for health workers cannot exist only during times of crisis, and through the sort of applause seen during the COVID-19 pandemic. It must come from fair pay so that women workers can live a decent life, free from chronic and normalised burnout.

The consequences of burnout are a driver of women's individual poor health and systemic in that burnout impacts on the services we depend on to improve women's health. Women like Rai leave their jobs. Women like the newly qualified nurses I met at the picket line start to think about what else they can do. Instead of investigating why women leave certain roles and the burdens that are placed on them, employers revert to stereotypical notions that women are not cut out for this work, can't handle the pressure, or were promoted too soon. This reinforces gender stereotypes of what senior leadership looks like and valorises the type of working environments that overlook the additional burdens women face in the workplace.

Health workers are fighting back on burnout and working conditions. Industrial action may result in a pay increase and improved working conditions for some health workers but not all. Nurses like those I met in London rejected the government's offer of a 5 per cent pay increase, but were unable to secure a mandate on further action as they did not reach the threshold of 50 per cent of all members of the Royal College of Nursing turning out to vote. In the end the 5 per cent pay offer was imposed on them, meaning nurses received a much smaller pay offer than the one they had hoped for. Effective industrial action depends on where in the world you work (in terms of both law around union membership and industrial action, and the culture of organised labour) and the power of your union and its members. If poor working conditions and burnout persist in health systems, there is a risk that gaps in health provision will increase as workers pursue other careers. This will be fine in a country like the UK. Rich countries will recruit from poorer countries to fill the gap. But this begs the question of what happens in poorer countries, where the gap in health workers is most acute and working conditions and pay are even worse. Who fills this gap? To answer this question, the next chapter looks at one of the most exploitative forms of women's labour in health: the millions of women working as volunteers, home-based carers, community health workers or semi-professional health workers. These workers are the ones counselling neighbours and friends and providing them with basic healthcare, educating their families and communities, and collecting data for major health security programmes. They are rarely paid. Without these women, multi-million-dollar foreign aid projects and domestic health systems would collapse. They are truly magnificent women, and are truly exploited by governments and donors who can and should recognise their work and pay them fairly.

9

The $1 Last Mile Health Workers

The first thing Lilian said to me when we met was that I would have to go and get changed. I thought I was interviewing her about her community health work in the villages surrounding Kisumu, the western hub of Kenya. Lilian had other ideas. I would not learn anything about what was happening with AIDS in Kenya from sitting in an office doing an interview in a dress. I got changed and got on a bike.

When we arrived in Kadibo thirty minutes later, I met Millicent, a community health worker whom Lilian had trained. It was 2005 and training of trainers was a big thing in the HIV/AIDS world. Lead trainers working for big international charities were training up health workers to do a range of care work in the community. This involved bathing people, fetching food and helping them prepare or eat it, delivering medicine, advising people of their rights and directing people to professional medical care if needed. Community health workers were often unpaid or only paid a per diem of around $1 a day, which they would use to buy food or supplies for the people they cared for. Despite receiving little or no pay, these volunteers were the backbone of the global response to HIV/AIDS. In the year that I met Lilian and Millicent, 2005,

HIV/AIDS was at the start of its financing boom, receiving US$4.8 billion in foreign aid to end the pandemic.[1] If you wanted to know what a policy set in the big decision-making centres such as Washington DC and Geneva looked like on the ground, it was here in Kadibo with women like Millicent: unpaid volunteers, almost always women, who were often HIV positive themselves.

Millicent told me she was pretty sure she was HIV positive but did not want to get tested. Her child was HIV positive and her husband was dying of AIDS. Not knowing her own status didn't stop her communicating government policy to the rest of her community: get tested, know your status, be faithful. Perhaps, like millions of women around the world, Millicent was too busy caring for others to look after her own health. No point wasting time getting tested for HIV when you are looking after family and neighbours dying from AIDS. Or perhaps she was scared, given what she saw her friends and neighbours go through living with the virus. I didn't ask, I just followed Millicent as she went about her work.

Millicent walked from home to home in a tightly clustered settlement of houses of roughly half a square kilometre. The homes were adobe houses, built from a combination of mud and straw, with two small rooms and no running water or electricity.

In the houses we visited, people were in their beds, looking sicker than anyone I have met before or since. Jennifer had terrible diarrhoea and could not sit up without the help of Millicent. She could only manage two spoonfuls of porridge a day and couldn't take water. Someone from a 'briefcase NGO' – a term for people who pretend to be NGOs to get aid money and then disappear – had 'signed her up' for treatment and never come back. All she had now was Millicent to care for her. Grace was lying on the floor in another house, mute, suffering from thrush, being taken care of by her mother and

Millicent. Her husband was next to her, also sick. He exposed himself to show me his herpes, saying 'Mzungu bring me dawa' (white person bring me medicine). I visited four different homes with the same problems: no will to test, no access to treatment, no means of getting to health facilities and a complete reliance on volunteers such as Millicent to care for them.

As we said our goodbyes to head off to the next community, Grace's mother ran towards me with a bag of rice. I was a guest and was not to leave empty handed. I tried to suggest that such a kind gift was unnecessary. Not wanting to offend, I explained I was staying in a hotel and did not have the means to cook the rice. Nevertheless, she persisted. Grace's mother could sense I was feeling overwhelmed by what I had seen, despite my efforts to put my best polite face on, so she forced the rice into my hand and then performed an elaborate running man dance move to cheer me up. She refused to stop until I smiled and laughed along, even mirroring her actions. It worked. Even where there is unnecessary death, there is a woman doing the running man to try and cheer people up.

Big international health programmes, with millions of dollars of investment, depend on women like Lilian, Millicent and Grace's mother to do the graft. These women are referred to as community health workers, home-based carers, peer educators, peer counsellors, extended family members, volunteers or just plain grandmothers in the official documentation that notes the important role they play. If you want to roll out a mass HIV-testing programme, a polio immunisation campaign or an Ebola behaviour-change programme, you need these women. No health policy in the world would work without them.

Community health workers are often the first to detect something happening in a community (the ones I've met can

also be terrific sources of local gossip) and are thus central to
reporting new viruses or disease outbreaks. They are also the
solution to the problem of 'the last mile' in global health. The
last mile refers to a situation where you have put all the appropriate public health measures in place, you have all the right
logistics frameworks, and medicines or vaccines are getting to
where they need to be, but still you cannot stop an outbreak,
complete an immunisation campaign or reach a specific community. The last mile is the stone in the shoe of public health
work, which is amplified in times of global health crisis. For
example, imagine you've spent two years dealing with a health
emergency that has devastated the health infrastructure and
economy of your country. You are so close to getting the cases
to zero, yet the odd case keeps popping up. You need local
intelligence on the ground to see where the cases are, why they
keep popping up, and stop them. To do this you need people
in these communities who you trust to tell you what's going
on. Not only that, they will fix it.

Community health workers are both the fixers and shit-
catchers in global health. They fix last-mile problems and
literally and figuratively catch the shit that governments and
health officials want to forget about or can't afford to pay for.
Community health workers are always the first to be called
when something needs fixing, but are always thought of last
in health policy and planning. They are mostly women and
rarely paid properly. Either they are labelled as volunteers and
not paid, or are paid a small amount of money to cover their
lunch and travel, or are paid a fee that barely meets even the
poorest of countries' minimum wage, or in a small number of
countries accredited and paid a basic wage. The Community
Health Impact Coalition, which tracks and advocates for community health-worker pay, suggests very few countries in the
world have up-to-date policies on community health workers,
and out of 245 countries in its database, only thirty-two have

both salaried and accredited community health workers.[2] One study on community health-worker pay suggested only 40 per cent globally were paid even a small amount, and in Africa, where community health workers fill multiple gaps in under-funded and under-staffed health systems, 85 per cent were unpaid.[3] The best paid and supported community health workers are in Brazil, Nigeria and South Africa, where they are paid $281–$472, $281 and $150–$290 per month respectively. This is most definitely the upper end of the salary scale for community health workers.[4] The majority in low-income countries, if paid at all, receive roughly $20 per month, or less than $1 a day.

When I met Millicent, Lilian and Grace's mother in 2005, billions of dollars were flowing to all sorts of people working in the AIDS response, from district council leaders to transport businesses and community groups, as well as the health sector and community health clinics who were rolling out new treatment for HIV and prevention guidelines. The money was paying for consultants, doctors, politicians, big international and small community charities, and researchers like me. Lilian was paid a small fee by the NGO she worked for, but the people doing the most work on the front line – workers like Millicent and Grace's mother – were getting nothing. The love and care of these women was sustaining billions of dollars' worth of aid projects and they were seeing pennies.

The reason women do this work is mixed. Love for community and family members is definitely a strong driver, either because it is a privilege to care for a sick friend or family member, or because if they don't do it no one else will. For some, the work is a form of prestige and recognition, especially if they are working for an international organisation. The esteem partly stems from the international actor recognising them and the work they do, but more important is the hope of more permanent, paid work, like an internship. Like many internships, permanent posts and better pay are always promised somewhere down the line but rarely come to anything. Finally, there is the more everyday version of why they do it: it's the only work they can get. While this work is rarely paid properly, a free T-shirt or a small $1 per diem is for some substantively better than nothing or going hungry through no work at all.

When asked about why these women are not paid, leaders of HIV/AIDS projects in national governments or the large foreign aid donors often acknowledge the important work they do, that maybe they are working on paying them, but more often deflect from the issue of payment. Aid donors and government officials insist that paying community health workers would be too difficult. It would be a logistical nightmare: you would need to identify who was doing what, what constitutes care and, my favourite rubbish excuse, paying people in the community is difficult because you have to handle large amounts of cash that may not get to where they need to go. This argument is used repeatedly *despite* cash transfers and mobile banking being advocated as solutions to poverty by the very same donors. When the logistics argument fails, the response falls back on the standard idea that women like Millicent do this work out of love for their community. And you do not need to be paid for doing the work of love and care.

The people who could do more for community health workers are well paid. Starting at the top, since 2018, the director-general of the WHO is paid US$239,755 with additional benefits linked to pension, travel, child education etc. Deputy director-generals are paid US$194,329 and the assistant director-generals US$176, 292. The most senior 'D2' salaries within the United Nations (apart from the secretary-general and assistant secretary-generals) start at $150,252 and go up to $181, 367, with additional benefits. Consultants paid to assess emergency plans, advise on the efficacy of disease surveillance and offer advice on what went wrong after the event are paid on average between $200 and $2,000 per day. If you work in private philanthropy you get paid even more. Jobs advertised in 2023 in gender equality and equality, diversity and inclusion in the Bill & Melinda Gates Foundation and the Wellcome Trust (which both do a lot of work around global health) offered a salary of $201,880–$374,920 and $256,500 respectively.

All of these roles will obviously be paid more than community health workers like Millicent living in rural East Africa. These people have advanced degrees, work under extreme pressure, have decades of experience and expertise, and much greater levels of responsibility. Their pay is an appropriate remuneration for their skill, responsibility and the requirements of the job. Most of the people I have met in these senior roles are incredibly hard working and most go beyond the specified hours of their contract (if such specification exists). They work for the love of the job and the importance they attribute to it. However, they are still paid. The love of their job does not equate to free or low-paid labour. It is not exploitative.

The most recent WHO data suggests there are 34,229,708 community health workers in the world.[5] Similarly to official numbers of paid health workers, 70 per cent of community health workers are women.[6] This number is taken from population censuses, employment surveys, health information systems and public payrolls. Therefore, it relies on people identifying, reporting and recording their activity as some kind of community health work. Lots of people doing health work in the community may not identify as such, so we can assume that the number of community health workers across the world is much higher than formal estimates suggest. The numbers don't cover the countless women like Millicent and Grace's mother, looking after extended family members, neighbours, educating and counselling as part of their every-day lives.

Given the scale of this work, it is likely that if you are a woman reading this, you are probably a community health worker. According to a study by researchers at the universities of Sheffield and Birmingham, if you are a woman living in the UK you have a 50 per cent chance of becoming a carer before you reach forty-six (for men it's fifty-seven).[7] You may not identify as such; you may even think it deeply problematic to do so, as what you perform is not necessarily work but something you do out of love for the people in your life. You don't mind caring for a loved one, as you love them and one day someone might have to care for you. Or maybe you know help is not coming from anywhere else, or the situation you're in has been assessed as not being bad enough to qualify for help. You just get on with it. But if you're shit-catching to make up for gaps in the health and social care system, or fixing problems as an afterthought, then you are part of a global phenomenon of women being exploited through their capacity and need to provide healthcare for loved ones or the communities in which they live.

SOPHIE: Who does the counting of new outbreaks and infections for the surveillance systems? More women or men?

KENNY: I can tell you it's like, we have about 90, 95, 98 per cent of women.

SOPHIE: Are they trained with additional skills to do this?

KENNY: Yes.

SOPHIE: Paid more?

KENNY: Erm, they don't get paid because I know a number of them are actually volunteers, yeah, but for a number of them it's pride.

Here we go again: another million-dollar health project depending on the free labour of women. My conversation at the start of 2020 was with Kenny, a data specialist working on the expansion of Sierra Leone's 'GIS Portal'. Geographic Information Systems (GIS) are a form of geospatial technology and are all the rage in public health planning. They became hugely popular after a succession of international health emergencies. The idea is that by mapping all sorts of information – number of health workers, reported outbreaks of new diseases or variants, travel and waiting times in health facilities, vaccine distribution – you can see how disease spreads, allowing decision makers to make 'precision' responses in specific geographic areas. Information and data are power in health: they are key to responding to outbreaks as soon as they occur, and tracking new threats by collating masses of data. Unsurprisingly, then, after Sierra Leone emerged from its Ebola crisis, all donor eyes were on developing data around people, mapping where and how they moved, and how they engaged with information.

GIS projects, such as the Sierra Leone one, are expensive and high profile. Sierra Leone's GIS Portal, for example, was supported by US$773,000 from the Bill & Melinda Gates Foundation.[8] They are part of even bigger-profile and highly funded projects around health emergency and pandemic preparedness. Since the early 2000s, an increase in health emergencies has led to greater funding and aid money towards detecting, responding to and preventing further health emergencies. You want to stop outbreaks becoming an emergency, and you definitely want to stop an emergency from becoming a pandemic. As part of this, donor countries gave substantial funds to poorer countries such as Sierra Leone to develop their surveillance systems and response capacity. The logic is all the global health security clichés: no one is safe until everyone is safe, diseases do not respect borders, and one country's response to an outbreak is only as strong as the weakest link in the chain. Prior to COVID-19, the idea was that to prevent the world from a pandemic, you had to invest in strengthening pandemic preparedness in poor countries. The more outbreaks occurred – H5N1, Ebola, Zika – the greater was the urgency to invest in the surveillance systems to detect them early. By 2020, the Health Emergencies Programme of the WHO had the fourth highest budget of the organisation, with $889 million allocated to it in the 2020–21 budget. By 2022–3 this had increased to the third highest budget within the organisation at $1.25 billion. GIS projects were both central to and some of the most expensive aspects of capacity building for global health security.

The women Kenny told me about underpinned all of this. They were the ones doing the counting of diseases per week in local communities in Sierra Leone. This is the bread-and-butter work of disease surveillance: to be able to identify emerging diseases and new threats, someone somewhere has to create the data that goes into the portal. It is skilled work that requires fostering trust between people living in the community and the health services, and identifying the correct symptoms.

One woman who had been trained to do this work was Fatima, a sixty-year-old grandmother from Kono, an, ahem, 'old woman', according to Kenny, who had never used a smartphone before. Kenny described how the woman, this data granny, was so proud of herself for using a smartphone, and how doing the training had improved her confidence. For Kenny, the work of data grannies was 'not much about money if you want to quantify it in monetary terms, but the joy alone that an old woman would have the opportunity to hold an android device, play with it, which we would just take for granted here, for them it's a big opportunity'.

This was not the first time someone leading a major foreign

aid initiative had mentioned to me the fundamental importance of grandmothers. People working in the international
world of health love grandmothers: if anyone could end AIDS,
or even bring about world peace, it would be the grandmothers of the world. They are the world's premier carers.
They could look after orphans, educate communities about
healthy behaviours, care for the sick and do data entry essential for disease surveillance. All for free! With all this praise
for grandmothers, only one prominent organisation – the
Stephen Lewis Foundation's Grandmothers to Grandmothers
Campaign – suggested that aid agencies, governments and
charities might pay them for trying to end the HIV/AIDS
pandemic.

The GIS project was definitely not aligned to this sort of
thinking. The whole system of global health security – de-
tecting and responding to outbreaks to keep us all safe – was
being underpinned by grandmothers working for free, all for
the 'joy' of holding a smartphone.

If you've ever had a smear test, you will know that as the
nurse inserts the speculum they will try and make polite
conversation to distract you. The nurse, Anne, who does my
smear tests left Sierra Leone during the civil war and has been
living in Britain and working in the NHS ever since. Hence
whenever the speculum goes in, polite conversation turns to
Sierra Leone gossip – mainly about ex-head of the military
and defence minister, Paolo Conteh. Anne returns to Sierra
Leone every year to see family and do some 'health work'
in the community. This is a common thing for many Sierra
Leoneans in the diaspora to do. Few return to Sierra Leone
to work permanently because the pay is too low, but they still
want to do something to help. Anne regularly stresses how
important this is to her and discusses the devastating state of
Sierra Leone's healthcare while brushing cells from my cervix.

Anne's position is part of a wider brain-drain phenomenon in healthcare work. This can be caused by war and conflict, as in the case of Anne, and the intersecting issue of poverty and low wages for health workers in poor countries. Many health workers earn better salaries abroad and send what they can in remittances to their wider families living back home. For poor countries, remittances can make up as much as 49.9 per cent of GDP in the case of Tonga, and 37.4 per cent in Lebanon.[9] Remittances can help health: they provide much-needed funds for family members to make out-of-pocket payments for their health needs. However, they can also exacerbate the problem of poor healthcare: it's one thing to be able to pay for health, it's another to have a workforce to provide it.

Health workers from poor countries sustain the health systems of rich ones. Since its creation at the end of the Second World War, the UK's NHS has been staffed by health professionals from Commonwealth countries who came to the UK to help rebuild the country and receive better wages. Attracting 'overseas health professionals' is what has kept the NHS workforce going, and this is very much the case today. As of 2022, the NHS was made up of a workforce from the UK (1,122,927), India (44,785), the Philippines (30,356), Nigeria (15,439), Ireland (13,762), Poland (10,836), Portugal (7,886), Italy (6,733), Pakistan (5,833), Romania (5,519), Zimbabwe (5,490), Spain (4,988), Ghana (4,581), Egypt (3,592) and Nepal (2,950).[10] Attracting world-class health professionals is an asset to a country like the UK, with an ageing population and increased care needs. And it is not just the UK. This pattern of health-worker migration from low to middle to high income, from Africa and Asia to Europe, Australia and North America happens across the world.

Some countries, such as the Philippines, see health-worker migration as a tool of economic growth. The country trains more health workers than it needs in order to export them to work in other countries. The funds that the workers send back to families in remittances make up a core of the country's GDP, and this is seen as a successful growth model. This model works for countries that have sufficient health-worker provision in their country. But then there is a country like Sierra Leone, which is at the other end of the scale.

One study in 2016 estimated that Sierra Leone had a combined workforce of one thousand doctors, nurses and midwives in the country; this translated to 1.4 per 10,000 population. To show how dire this shortage is, in comparison, England's health workforce is made up of 1.5 million people (1.2 million full time); this in turn equates to 265.3 health workers per 10,000 population.[11] Such a health-worker shortage would be bad in any country, but this shortage is in a country that regularly tops the chart of worst health outcomes, notably the highest rates of maternal mortality in the world. The problem with the brain drain of medical professionals is that a country like Sierra Leone will always be playing an impossible game of catch up. First, the country has to hold on to the medical professionals it has. This is not easy when they are overworked, undervalued, often not paid on time and working in poor conditions that often lack basic medical supplies. Second, training of medical professionals takes time and investment, both in short supply in low-income settings. Third, the salaries paid to professionals have to compete with salaries paid in higher income states. This is a huge distortion to levels of pay in the economy. It also rests on richer countries in turn not increasing salary levels to attract health workers. The gap potentially gets bigger.

And who fills the gap that's left in the health sector in the interim? Low and/or unpaid female community health workers.

According to Sierra Leone's 'Basic Package of Essential Health Services', 'Community Health Workers are the main staffing cadre at community level', but they are not really paid. They receive $13.50 a month plus a 'small allocation' for travel expenses, which brings the total up to $14. This is significantly less than the *minimum* wage of $40 a month set by the Sierra Leone government. There are 13,000 known community health workers who have had the requisite ten-day government training to do their job. There are many more unknown who don't even get paid $13.50 a month. According to the Sierra Leone government and the WHO's African office, 48 per cent of health workers in Sierra Leone are unsalaried.[12]

With stopgaps come problems. Some health activists in Sierra Leone warned me that the gaps community health workers filled were so big that they were engaged in work that was beyond them. For example, one health researcher explained to me that community health workers were sometimes the only healthcare professional in peripheral health units – the first tier of health provision for many Sierra Leoneans. As a result, sometimes they tried to do things that were way beyond their skillset, training or knowledge, such as delivering babies. The health researcher continued, 'They don't have the skills to even identify that I need to refer her now, and by the time they realise oh I need to refer, you know it's at the later stage and sometimes they die in the ambulance or when they get to hospital.' The problem of community health workers filling a gap is that they are not only being exploited, but they are not fit to fill the gap. Trying their best in a difficult situation, such as a complicated birth, can have fatal consequences.

The Sierra Leone government, the donors that support the health sector and the WHO all know that community health-worker pay and dependency is a huge problem in poor countries. The issue is too big to ignore and it's set to get worse. Remember the shocking statistic from the last chapter: the WHO predicts a shortfall of 18 million health workers by 2030.[13] Poor countries will bear the brunt of this shortfall.

Women in poor countries will bear the brunt of this shortfall: they'll be the ones expected to fill the growing gap, still unpaid and exploited for their labour.

The worst thing about knowing and acknowledging the role of community health workers and not paying them, is there *are* models of how this can be done effectively. Advocates of paying community health workers all point to countries such as Brazil, Bangladesh, Ethiopia and, of course, Rwanda.[14] Advocates such as the Community Health Impact Coalition provide clear resources on how to pay community health workers. Health economists interested in this work are great at proposing models of payment and making the investment case. The Women's Budget Group, for example, calculated that every 2 per cent of GDP invested in the care sector generated employment increases of between 1.2 and 3.2 per cent, depending on the country: more jobs creates more tax revenue, thus the caring economy is a money maker for governments.[15] The investment money has to come from somewhere, but when governments need to find money for wars, building walls and bailing out banks, they do. Similarly, when donors need to pay for major health security surveillance systems, they find funds for expensive tech, but never the relatively cheap and affordable work of people doing the last mile. The evidence of how and why to do it is there. Not paying community health workers and carers is a political choice.

If women's health is at the centre of attention in global politics, it is women themselves who are at the centre of delivering the ambitious health targets and foreign aid programmes. As I've shown in Part 2 of this book, their labour is exploited for little or no pay, and their bodies are abused and sexually exploited by men running the programmes meant to save lives. The most vulnerable women in the world are unable to seek out healthcare from medical charities without their stories being used to attract money. The most sickening part of this exploitation is that it is silenced and made invisible through stigma, shame, love and the idea that any woman who speaks out about her exploitation threatens the greater good of health for all.

When women are exploited and their health needs are not met, policy-makers and practitioners often reach for SOS! – the same old solutions: get more women into leadership positions, get the gender experts in and get better data to prove the problem exists and how much it will cost to do something about it. However, as the final part of this book suggests, these common solutions to old problems are not the magic bullet we want them to be, especially when they are subject to different versions of the same bias and inequality we have seen thus far.

Part 3

SOS!
(Same Old Solutions)

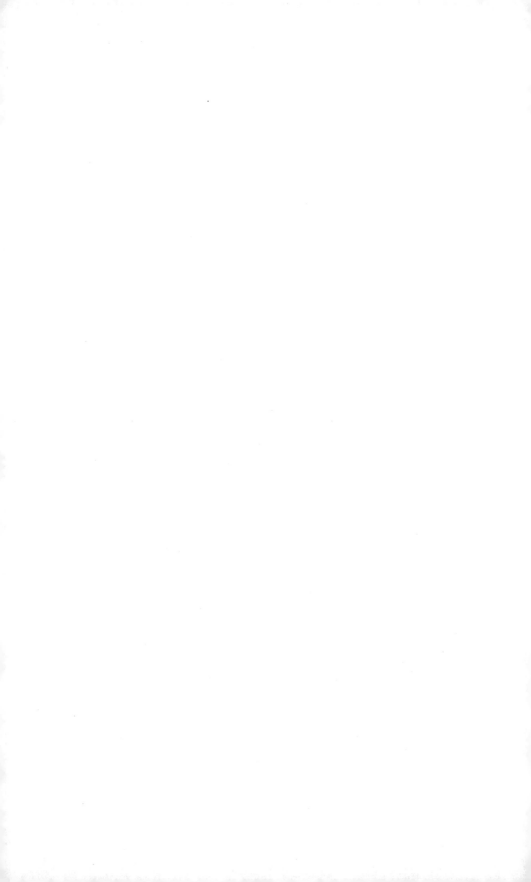

10

Women Leaders and the Most Qualified Candidate

Every third week of September, all the member states of the world converge on New York City for the gathering of the General Assembly. It is the annual UN jamboree where state delegations press the flesh, do deals, have informal one-on-one meetings, take to the podium to state their intent for the world and clog up the traffic of midtown Manhattan. In September 2010, Melinda French Gates, one of the world's biggest philanthropists, took to the General Assembly's green marble podium. Reading from a well-rehearsed script, French Gates spoke of optimism and all lives having equal value as a way of showing her commitment to the UN Global Strategy on Women's, Children's and Adolescents' Health, 'Every Woman, Every Child', announced by UN secretary-general, Ban Ki-moon that week. French Gates and the foundation she founded with her husband, Bill Gates of Microsoft, would pledge $1.5 billion to women and children's health, nutrition and family planning over a five-year period.[1] This was a game-changing amount of funds for women's health. French Gates wasn't just talking about inspiration and optimism, she was leading this change and putting the foundation's money where her mouth was.

French Gates is one of the examples men give me when I question the lack of female leadership and representation in health around the world. She is one of the most powerful women in the world. You may be less familiar with her name than that of her ex-husband Bill, but make no mistake: if you are interested in power in women's health, you should know about Melinda. The Bill & Melinda Gates Foundation funds every aspect of global health, including all the major UN bodies that work on health. After the US government, the foundation is the second biggest donor to the WHO. It gives millions of dollars to university research programmes throughout the world. It supports media outlets, from the *Guardian* to the Bureau of Investigative Journalism, to report on and showcase different issues of international development and global health. Name any project related to health around the world and chances are the foundation will be involved somehow. As of 2022, the foundation has spent $71.4 billion in grant payments in 144 countries, and it only has to answer to eight people – its board of trustees (two of whom are Bill and Melinda). French Gates is considerably more powerful than an elected world leader because of her money, networks, foundation, ex-husband and a profile that is not dependent on electoral votes or the interests of member state allies and enemies. French Gates can influence world decisions and use her money to advance her interests for as long as the money lasts. She has the ear of world leaders, she can give speeches on all the major world stages – the UN in New York, the World Economic Forum in Davos, the World Health Assembly in Geneva. If French Gates wants to prioritise women's maternal health, this will become a priority in the world. She is not just one of the most powerful women in the world: she is one of the most powerful people in the world.

Health cannot have a female leadership problem because

the biggest philanthropist in global health is a woman who is using her power to advance women's health and, to top that, in the early 2020s most of the UN health leaders were black women from middle-income countries. The other names I hear when I am complaining about the paucity of women leaders are of ex-director-generals of the WHO, Gro Harlem Brundtland and Margaret Chan, and heads of the other major health agencies, as of 2023: Winnie Byanyima (UNAIDS), Natalia Kanem (UNFPA), Sima Sami Bahous and her predecessor Phumzile Mlambo-Ngcuka (UN Women).

If you need to see it to be it then these women are an inspiration to girls and women around the world. These women reflect the 70 per cent of women in the global health workforce (although, other than Chan and Kanem, none of them have worked in front-line health work). They are at the top of their professions, taking on diverse portfolios, investing and tracking billions of dollars, responding to major emergencies and managing the highest level of global bickering, lies and gossip, which makes up modern international relations. If you were to look at this group of women you would think things had moved on – that in 2023 women ruled the world, or at least the patch of women's health in the world.

But you'd be wrong.

According to the 2022 report of the research group Global Health 50/50, women hold 40 per cent of board seats of the most influential public and private health organisations in the world.[2] Only 9 per cent of these seats are held by women from low- and middle-income countries, and only 1 per cent of seats are occupied by women from low-income countries. Fifty-eight per cent of the organisations reviewed in the study have never had a female CEO, and 51 per cent have never had a female chair of the board. Those responsible for health around the world are not the Melindas and Winnies, they are the Bills, Michels and Richards (there are a lot of Richards).

The system of representation in health around the world is upside down. As Part 2 of this book showed, and advocacy organisation Women in Global Health put it, the world's healthcare is 'delivered by women, led by men'. Hence, when thinking about how to fix the problems of women's health, one of the go-to same old solutions – SOS! – is to see greater representation of women at the top. Leadership matters, as women's health advocate Joia Crear Perry of the Black Mamas Matter Alliance told me: 'I want to be clear, the things you need are actual power, decision-making, budget.' Without power, decision-making and budget, you can't shift the dial on paying community health workers, ensuring decent working conditions for health workers, protecting health facilities in conflict or increasing comprehensive sexual health allocations (I could go on). Women won't necessarily make better leaders than men in health, but given the gross misrepresentation and mess we're already in with women's health, it can't hurt to try. Which is why women's leadership becomes such a prominent SOS!

The problem, however, is women leaders in the health sector face much of the same discrimination you're probably already familiar with – pay inequality, under-promotion, alpha males, the Ginger Rogers 'backwards in heels' effect – referring to the American entertainer Ginger Rogers, who had to do everything her dance partner Fred Astaire did, but backwards and in high heels – and of course your views and contributions being overlooked next to your male partner (admit it, before you read the start of this chapter, you knew more about Bill than Melinda). You might think that women being the majority of workers in health with role models like French Gates and Byanyima would help. But no. Women's majority status can be used to deflect questions of representation – women are everywhere so of course they are represented! If there is a problem in leadership it is not because of a pipeline problem, it is an individual confidence problem – women are everywhere, they just need to put themselves forward! To understand how this works, I want to introduce you to two of the most qualified candidates in women's health.

While movies depict the world of international affairs as fast-paced meetings of suited or uniformed men in glass boxes or underground bunkers with the occasional flag or government crest, the reality of these spaces tends to be to row after row of plain walls with grey dividers between desks. This is especially the case at the offices of the biggest international development agency in the world, the World Bank. It is impossible not to get lost looking for someone in the World Bank; once you're past the security door, every desk looks the same.

When I eventually found the office of the leader of the World Bank's HIV/AIDS programme in 2006, I was briefly taken aback. Here was the colour. Here were carpets with different shapes and colours of condoms from around the world. I was in the World Bank, but I was not in the usual World Bank office, and was clearly dealing with a different character than all the health economists I'd previously met.

Debrework Zewdie was as much of an anomaly as her condom carpets. She was a Black Ethiopian woman, but even more rare to the Bank: she was not an economist. The Bank fames itself as having the most PhDs of any major organisation, and she definitely had one of those, but it was in clinical immunology rather than development economics. Zewdie had come to the Bank's Human Development department in 1994 after working for USAID in Kenya. This was the beginning of a time of great change at the Bank. The incoming president, James Wolfensohn (World Bank president, 1995–2005), was about to introduce his programme to make the Bank more encompassing of a broader range of development issues and ways of working. As I mentioned in Chapter 2, the Bank had

undergone twenty years of criticism from all member states –
rich and poor – about the way it lent poor countries money
and told them what to do, with at times the result of making
poor countries worse off after years of 'support'. The Bank in
the mid-1990s therefore faced a challenge: adapt or die. The
Bank chose to adapt – ish. Part of the adaptation was to see
what crises were really affecting poor countries. The big one
was AIDS and Zewdie was at the heart of it.

When I first met Zewdie in 2006, I was already aware of her
impact on women's health. While researching my PhD on the
politics of HIV/AIDS, her name kept coming up as the woman
who changed the game on funding to AIDS programmes, not
just in the World Bank, but across the aid sector. I had heard
a lot of remarkable stories about key individuals in the fight to
get the world to take notice of the HIV/AIDS crisis, but nearly
all of them had been about men. The Peters, the Richards and
the Pauls. Here was a Debrework.

The story of what Zewdie managed to achieve with the
HIV/AIDS project is pretty remarkable. She set up the world's
first major multilateral funding project for HIV/AIDS. She
was the first person to get a pledge for AIDS that was in the
billions rather than the millions of dollars. She got the biggest
global aid agency in the world to change how it worked, who
it funded and what it funded. What is doubly impressive is
that once she was done with the Bank, she went to the new
AIDS funder on the block – the Global Fund to Fight AIDS,
Tuberculosis and Malaria – and did it all over again.

What is perhaps the most impressive thing about Zewdie is
not what she did but how she did it. She came to work on the
HIV/AIDS project because of an opportunity. Her boss had to
read the latest book on development economics and, like many
bosses, didn't have time, so asked her to do it. Being diligent,
she did. Recognising her talent, her boss then insisted that
as she had read the book and worked in Africa, she be in all

meetings on AIDS and offer insight into what the Bank should be doing about a disease that was killing in the millions.

At the time, the Bank was dead set against this. Giving money to a health issue? That was not the sort of macro-economic thinking the Bank was used to. They wanted major structural transformation of poor countries' economies. HIV/AIDS was not a part of that. On the other side, many public health people were against the Bank becoming involved with health issues because they thought that past World Bank interventions had transformed economies in such a way as to devastate public health systems in poor countries.

Zewdie had to convince the Bank that this was what they should do, and to convince her peers that she was not a sell-out by working with the Bank. She started by building the evidence. She convened a group of scientists and experts to meet at the Bank and show the economists the evidence of the impact of AIDS on life expectancy, economic growth and all manner of social ills, from early school dropouts to millions of orphans and vulnerable children. She, in her own words, 'had to beg and cry and all kinds of things to get the Vice President for the Africa region and the Vice President for Human Development to chair that half day meeting'. The trick, knowing the vice president for Africa was Zimbabwean, was to show what would happen in Zimbabwe specifically. It worked. He attended and was shocked by the evidence. When they asked what could be done, she replied simply, 'You give us money.'

Zewdie wanted a grant, not a loan, for countries, so that they would not find themselves in crippling debt for trying to sort out the AIDS crisis. The first committee she attended brushed it aside. Upset, she left the committee room and walked around Washington DC for hours before heading home. She got home to an answering machine full of urgent messages. The vice president had been looking for her. He had even come up from the fifth to the eighth floor. This was unheard of. She was summoned to see him the next day. However, once back in the office she stayed put, because she was worried she would break down if he said no. Upset or not, it takes some cajones not to go and see a big boss when they ask to see you. He sent his assistant back up to the eighth floor to get her.

As Zewdie told me, 'I went and sat down and he said, "What do you want?" And they gave me everything I asked: 500 million dollars.'

The first US$500 million was agreed in May 2000, on condition that she bring two completed pilot projects to the Bank board in September. The usual emergency Bank project at the time would be given six months, but she was given three. She delivered by September and was immediately given an additional US$500 million to continue.

The first billion-dollar HIV/AIDS project was born.

Zewdie is exactly what the world needs more of. She typifies the promise of female leaders who get shit done. She stands out in a world of men called Richard, Peter and Paul as a Black female senior leader born in a middle-income country. She used male allies, adapted her practice and approach, and delivered the goods to effect change. She exhibited just the sort of leadership that Facebook chief operating officer Sheryl Sandberg was talking about when she wrote her bestselling book *Lean In*: she got a powerful male patron, took risks by stepping across the 'jungle gym' from public health to the world of development economics, and did it all with good humour. She embodies 'the moment of lift' that Melinda French Gates talks about when she discusses women's empowerment throughout the world. She showed exactly what a woman could achieve in a position of power.

But then there is the other reading of Zewdie's story. The

one where she had to work under a shorter time period to get her project approved. She had to show exceptional skill to be taken seriously. The whole thing relied on the luck and patronage of her professional relationships with male colleagues. And she was paid *much less* than men when she started at the World Bank. When I asked why she told me, 'Because I was coming from a developing country, because I didn't know the mechanics of the World Bank, I was hired at a much lower level and salary than somebody who had the exact same kind of credentials.' It does not matter how influential and effective Zewdie was: she fitted the pay gap mould. In one joint study by the WHO and the ILO on health-worker pay in fifty-four countries, women were on average paid 20 per cent less than men.[3]

Pay is an important issue when it comes to representation. Pay can be a proxy for value and seniority. If women are paid less because of the gender pay gap this undermines their value and can impact on their access to senior leadership positions. For example, one form of hidden bias on selection committees (of any level, but this is acute for leadership roles) is assessing candidates based on their current salary. The gender pay gap across the health sector means women are penalised twice, first by getting paid less than men for doing the same work, and second, when we go for other jobs or opportunities our relative low pay infers a lower status in comparison to our better-paid male colleagues.[4] Pay is important: unless women are paid equally to men, their leadership will not be viewed as equal by either their peers or even themselves. If you pay a woman leader less, you are saying she's worth less. Women in turn may believe in the value pay puts on them and internalise a sense that they have less value, or skill to lead. You therefore cannot address the question of women's leadership and representation within global health without addressing their pay.

Zewdie is not alone. Across health, women leaders face

discrimination and tactics to discredit their work or are asked to do more work to justify the change they want to see, all while being paid less. This is often referred to as the Ginger Rogers effect. For example, when ex-BBC journalist Carrie Gracie sued the BBC for pay discrimination after finding out that she was paid less as China editor than her male counter-parts as Europe and US editors, she quoted the Ginger Rogers effect. Gracie agreed to take the job if she was paid the same as the other editors. She was not, despite being made to believe she was. All three roles had the same status in terms of geo-political importance, but she was doing the job in Mandarin under the gaze of an authoritarian regime watching her every move – same work, but backwards in heels. What she found when she challenged the pay disparity was that it got personal: people started to suggest she was somehow less qualified for the position.

Women in leadership in global health face a similar bind. To advance, they have to be Ginger Rogers and are expected to do more for less. But when they want to advance or push for pay equality they are discredited as less qualified. It does not matter how qualified or how much merit or expertise a woman has, being deemed the most qualified often depends on whether you are a man and, as I set out below, who you know.

'It is a great diplomatic victory and the recognition of Congolese competence on a world scale: Doctor Jean Kaseya takes the head of the CDC.'[5]

So began the press release from the office of the president of the DRC, President Félix-Antoine Tshisekedi Tshilombo, following the announcement of the new director-general of Africa CDC (Centres for Disease Control and Prevention) as Dr Jean Kaseya, a male medical doctor from the DRC. The president was correct: beating 180 candidates and winning the largest percentage of votes from member states of the African Union to land the top job *is* a diplomatic victory. Africa CDC is a significant political actor on health and foreign aid issues in the world. It is responsible for the African continent's health-emergency planning and preparation, and is a lead actor in developing the African Union's vision for a more sustainable solution to Africa's health problems, including the African Union's ambitious strategy to set up vaccine manufacturing hubs across the continent. Africa CDC is not *just* crucial for the health and well-being of Africans, but for the health of the world because Africa is a region where new outbreaks of major diseases occur, and all the major health players pump money into and extract knowledge from it. The appointment of the new director came at a critical time in which the African Union and various foreign aid donors were looking to boost the work of the organisation. To get your man in the leadership position is a good strategic move.

To find the right person for the job, a committee made up of health ministers from the region whittled down 180 candidates to two finalists. They interviewed the finalists and put forward the recommended final candidate to the African Union heads of state. The heads of state then ratified the candidate recommended by the committee. This was despite three countries requesting further debate on the issue.[6] Member states wanted additional time to scrutinise the candidates, recognising that not all heads of state had attended the final meeting, preferring to send their deputies or representatives, and because those who were in attendance and requested additional time for debate were ignored. Fair processes are important to any job selection, be it the front desk receptionist or the head of Africa CDC.[7]

The successful candidate, Kaseya, had worked for UNICEF for nine years; Gavi, the Vaccine Alliance (the world's main vaccine organisation) for two years; as senior country director for ex-US president Bill Clinton's the Clinton Health Access Initiative; the Bill & Melinda Gates Foundation for some months; and crucially as senior advisor to the president and routine immunisation officer in the DRC.[8] The second of the two candidates, Dr Magda Robalo Correia e Silva was also a medical doctor, but with an added postgraduate diploma in public health and tropical medicine and an MSc in epidemiology. She had far more extensive experience of working in global health, having worked as: chair of the Ethics and Governance Committee of the Global Fund to Fight AIDS, Tuberculosis and Malaria; member of the WHO Global Expert Panel on Health Emergency and Risk Management; an employee of the WHO for over twenty years with roles including director of communicable diseases, malaria regional advisor, country representative to Ghana, and other positions. On the domestic front, she was minister of public health in Guinea-Bissau, where she co-ordinated the country's response to COVID-19. Finally, she had set up the Institute for Global Health and Development, the first hepatitis prevention and control programme in all of Africa, and numerous emergency and disaster response initiatives, and is a mentor of the Kofi Annan Global Health Leadership Programme of Africa CDC.[9]

A large number of member states agreed that Robalo was by far the most qualified candidate.[10] But Kaseya got the job because the one thing he had that she didn't was presidential support. DRC President Félix Tshisekedi boasted about the 'long secret diplomatic battle waged for 6 months' and his 'great diplomatic victory by snatching this post'. The press release missed out President Tshisekedi's other role as a UN HeForShe Champion, where men pledge their commitment to advancing women and gender equality rather than snatching posts away from more qualified women.[11] Kaseya didn't succeed just because he had a HeForShe Champion fighting his diplomacy battle to get the right man in the job; it was also because he had the backing of his government. Robalo did not. The president of Guinea-Bissau was keen to let all the other African leaders know that Guinea-Bissau did not have an official candidate. It was a power play, because he did not want a leader from his country occupying a more powerful role than his in African affairs, and especially not a woman. Robalo not only had to compete with the diplomatic game of getting member states to back her; she also had to deal with the most difficult of challenges: the male ego. As Robalo stated in her letter to the African Union when she found out what had happened, there was no requirement for a candidate to be backed by their head of state. But when it came down to it, merit, experience and being the best qualified person for the job did not get Kaseya the position: it was the politics.

The appointment of director of Africa CDC is no different to very senior leadership appointments in all international organisations. No candidate can ever be successful without the backing of major member states and intense diplomacy to win enough votes to be appointed to the position. While experts and committees can affect who is on the shortlist and who is supported, it is member states who have the final decision. These are supposed to be neutral, technical appointments, but they are imbued with international relations between states. It is telling, for example, that the only head of state to speak out against the circumstances of Kaseya's appointment to Africa CDC was Paul Kagame, president of Rwanda, who has tense relations with the DRC.

While networks and diplomacy apply to both men and women seeking leadership positions, such practices put women at a particular disadvantage. One study of medical practitioners published in the *Lancet* noted the importance of networking for career progression, and that despite the best attempts made by women to access these networks, 'Women were often excluded from networking activities dominated by men.'[12] This maps onto common experiences of women in many different professions who attempt to build networks but often find themselves excluded or overlooked in favour of men. On the world stage, you can amplify this exclusion further: the practice of foreign policy and international diplomacy is dominated by men, and the majority of world leaders are men. Women are only put forward by heads of state for such roles if the governments of countries believe women belong in foreign policy, and many governments around the world do not. Women who break through these male-dominated barriers to work in foreign policy and diplomacy are often highly effective, but still end up writing memoirs as to why they never belonged or were never expected to be there in the first place.

Zewdie recognised the importance of networks in international diplomacy. Seeing how the men went on golf trips, and felt more comfortable reaching out for advice from other men, she developed her own networks with women from the World Bank, particularly with more junior women at earlier stages of their career. She also developed relationships with member state governments and men working in the Bank. Her approach was to build mentorship and support for other women, while cultivating male allyship. Male allies, #heforshe, all amount to the same thing: men supporting women and addressing discrimination and inequalities women face. For women in leadership this means supporting women to become leaders, building networks around a woman leader, and sometimes stepping aside. Women need a patron to become leaders. The risk of having a patron is that women become the client. If the patron does you a favour and supports your candidacy for a leading position, you owe them as the client. This both accentuates their power as a patron, and women's dependency on powerful men to get ahead. It is hardly smashing the glass ceiling, rather being in constant debt to the men who gave you the hammer.

Robalo follows a long line of women in politics and international relations who should have got the job over the man. She is the Hillary Rodham Clinton of the health world: decades of experience and knowledge with a clear plan. A position as head of a regional health body is, of course, different from being the president of the US, where individual voters and party politics play a big role. It is also different for an important reason: health is supposed to prioritise science and evidence over all else. This should also apply to assessing who is the most qualified candidate for a role. But, yet again, health is not about science but international politics, and so ultimately the most qualified candidate is a political not scientific calculation in which women are always at a disadvantage.

Zewdie retired from international service and took up visiting professorships at the City University of New York (CUNY) and Harvard, where she teaches leadership in public health. Like Robalo, she did make a bid for some of the top jobs in global health, most notably the executive director of UNAIDS, but as many other women have found, the men at the time apparently had more qualifications and experience (they didn't). People who worked in the global health sector know of her contribution to ending HIV/AIDS; however, her name is perhaps less familiar than her male contemporaries who went on to head major UN and funding organisations, to write autobiographies and to appear on media shows such as the BBC's *Desert Island Discs* (see, for example, Peter Piot, ex-UNAIDS and former director of the London School of Hygiene and Tropical Medicine, and Jeremy Farrar, ex-director of the Wellcome Trust). But her legacy in changing the landscape of HIV/AIDS financing and governance while dancing backwards in heels for less money is still felt in contemporary health projects.

The expectation that all women have to be more Zewdie or

Robolo puts a lot of pressure on women in leadership positions: they not only have to excel in a role while getting paid less, there is an expectation that they will advance change for women and gender equality, regardless of whether they want to or not, all in addition to their stated job. Women should not be seen as the solution to systemic inequalities. Women should not be the SOS! to all problems and inequalities in the world. These inequalities are bigger than individual women. This type of what bell hooks calls 'faux feminism'[13] puts all the onus on the individual to effect change, not the perpetrator of the problem – the sexist, racist and elitist institutions in which women work. And it favours women tweaking institutions and working within them rather than enacting wholesale, widespread change. Not only does this limit change, but it creates a reversal in feminist gains, as such faux feminism (also sometimes called feminism-lite or corporate feminism) becomes a smokescreen for wider change. It gives health providers and institutions a handy feminism-lite solution to their gender equality problems: just get women to try harder and apply themselves more. And it strips away the wider politics of *how* people get to these positions: as if they get to them through merit and hard work. No one becomes a senior leader through merit and hard work alone, especially in the international community. It is a con to think that anyone, especially women operating in spaces dominated by men, can overcome structures of inequality to gain positions of power without political support of some kind.

The trick that all working women come to realise at some point in their professional lives is you can work as hard as you can, do all the networking and be more than qualified for the job, but you will never be seen as the most qualified candidate. And, to top it off, if you do get to the top as a woman you will be expected to be the SOS! – to solve all the problems of your employer.

*

Health sectors around the world pose one of the starkest absurdities of gender inequality. Here is a sector staffed by women, whose work is determined almost entirely by men. The people making decisions about women's health are not only male world leaders intent on exploiting women's health for votes, it is also men at the top of the organisations that direct funding to health, men who decide which research counts as important and men who push and pull member states to fall in with global priorities. When extremely qualified women put themselves forward for leadership positions, the most qualified male candidate gets the job. The evidence and meritocracy of science goes out of the window when a successful woman steps up to lead.

This leads us to the next SOS! If the institutions themselves are sexist and don't understand gender equality, and there are no women leaders to fix the problem for you, bring in the gender experts.

11

Call (and Ignore) the Gender Expert

As a senior African woman with decades of expertise on gender and health, Faith knew she had to step up and speak out when Sierra Leone faced one of the worst Ebola outbreaks in history in 2014/16. She had worked in the capital Freetown as a gender expert in the UN delegation for nearly a decade, and across Africa for many more years. She had witnessed the ongoing impact of sexual violence against women during Sierra Leone's civil war. She had worked with colleagues to combat one of the most taboo subjects in West Africa, FGM, and had gone through successive plans, funding commitments and politicians' pledges to do something (and always something different) to reduce the high levels of maternal mortality in the country. More than that, she always had one foot in the communities she worked in. To be good at her job within the UN, no matter how senior her status, Faith had to be across the everyday issues women in Sierra Leone were facing. Not only that, she had to know how to communicate these issues to politicians and international donors for them to be taken seriously. Faith knew when and how to shout extra loud. She was no stranger to emergencies or staring down male colleagues when they didn't want to hear what she had to say. For her, working in Sierra Leone and seeing the changes that had been made after the civil war had been a real privilege. Her story is one of the power of gender experts as an SOS! for improving women's health. When you can't get a woman to lead an organisation and change it, you can get a gender expert to flag – and, if necessary, shout about – the issues that matter and tell you what to do about them.

As soon as Ebola broke out, Faith and her team hit the ground to find out how the outbreak was affecting women. Her networks in the sector were starting to identify worrying trends: sexual violence in quarantines, abuse by security personnel enforcing curfews, women staying away from hospital to give birth, and dying as a consequence, an increase in intimate-partner violence, and stigma towards female nurses and community health workers. Faith knew this risked becoming a tidal wave of abuse, burden and poor health for women. Women were not safe in quarantines. Women needed help getting food and supplies for their families. Women needed PPE that fitted them in order to go door to door to test and inform their neighbours and friends of the risks. As a precursor of what was to come for women around the world during the COVID-19 pandemic in 2020, women were on the front line and needed help.

Faith warned the leaders of the Ebola response. It was not Ebola that was the threat to women, it was how the response to Ebola risked women's lives. Unless help was concentrated on women, the fight against Ebola would not be won, and any advances the country had made on gender equality would be set back by decades. The stakes were that high.

She raised the flag.

And the response?

'Ah, you're always going on about women, everybody is dying ... You know everybody is dying, this is an emergency, we have no time for that.'

This is an emergency, we have no time for that.

This was not the first time Faith had heard such a response. She was told to get additional evidence. She got it. One member of the response team discredited her evidence as 'not scientific'. She got more scientific data. She went back to the leaders again.

In front of the most senior members of the Sierra Leone military, the government and major international donors, Faith calmly set out the differing – and worse – impact Ebola was having on women than on men. More women were dying than men. More women were vulnerable as front-line health workers. Women were being put at risk due to public health measures such as curfews and quarantines. And if unchecked, the secondary threats to women's health that had plagued Sierra Leone for decades – notably unsafe childbirth, FGM, lack of breast cancer screening – would be bigger than the threat of Ebola.

This time no one dismissed the evidence. Instead, there was a deadly silence. Everyone in the room realised two things: first that by now it was probably too late – the damage to women had already been done; second, that they had missed a trick all along – to beat this thing they would need to engage women and bring them on board. By dismissing women's needs, they were overlooking one of the most powerful resources they had: a cadre of women who had the trust of their families and communities to carry the message of what to do to keep safe, to report back what was happening in the communities to the central command structures, and to pick up any slack in the system. As soon as the women were seen as useful, they mattered.

The silence was so tense that Faith made a joke to ease the atmosphere. She had raised the flag, been dismissed, raised the flag again and was now trying to make everyone feel better about the situation. Domestic violence had skyrocketed, more women *did* die from pregnancy-related complications than Ebola,[1] with a 34 per cent increase in maternal mortality (based on data captured in clinics) and a 24 per cent increase in stillbirths. Teenage pregnancy had shot up in a country that already held the record for all-time highs for teen pregnancy in the world. To top it off, when Ebola was in retreat and the schools reopened, pregnant girls were not allowed to return as the government thought their pregnancy would prevent them from learning, cause them to be bullied, and inspire others to become pregnant. It was as if no one had learned anything from listening to the gender experts.

Gender experts are a great SOS! to the problem of women's poor health; they are good at identifying and flagging issues and often, like Faith, have strong links and networks to women most in need and the organisations that help them. Gender experts working within organisations are slightly different from women's health specialists. These experts look at how the gendered determinants of health are being addressed; the impacts of health emergencies and how issues affect different genders, inclusive of people with diverse gender identities; how gender is accounted for in institutional strategies, planning and budgeting; and wider gender equality practices within the institution. A lot of their work overlaps with women in health work, but they are not women's health specialists akin to, say, an obstetrician. They tend to have social sciences or humanities degrees and experience rather than science or medical backgrounds. This is an asset – they know their gender politics – but can also be a detriment, as like Faith, they and the issues they raise can be seen among health colleagues as secondary to the primacy of science and medicine. Their job is to get institutions to take gender inequality seriously in how it impacts on health outcomes and unnecessary deaths. It is to be the flagbearer of gender equality – equality between men, women and gender-diverse people – and to hold people to account when they don't meet the mark.

Gender experts are often few and far between in health settings (this is why I am quite vague about the background and roles of the gender experts in this chapter: given how tough and at times sensitive their job is I don't want to identify them), and they need to be listened to and believed in order to create change. More often, like Faith, they are overworked and discredited. Like other women working in the health sector in Part 2, the work of gender experts is often undermined because it is women's work, only relevant when it is seen by the powers that be to have value for the rest of society. This is the bind gender experts face as part of the SOS! to improve women's health: they know how valuable and essential their work is, but also that they will be overworked, ignored until it is too late and undervalued. As I will explore in this chapter, to navigate the world of a gender expert in health, you don't just need feminist persistence and energy, but frameworks, young people and, crucially, humour. And you need people to listen.

Jane is a gender expert who comes from the activist and NGO world. She has built up decades of expertise working in the NGO sector and the UN. When I spoke to her, she had been working as a senior gender expert in a major UN health agency for a year and a half. Prior to getting the job, she thought she knew the score. Gender work was always difficult, and would always risk backlash, but this was a UN agency that had high-lighted a gender-focused approach to its work. It would be a challenging job, but here was an opportunity, not a risk. She would be at the forefront of driving their strategy forward and building best practice for other UN agencies to learn from. She would work side by side with the executive director. The executive director was a vocal feminist: she imagined their leadership would be different from the usual UN boss. Like many, she believed it was the UN where you could make the big changes.

Her hopes were quickly dashed. Her first year in the job was a wake-up call as to the reality of being the main gender expert. The constant demands on her time and others questioning her role started to exhaust her. The gender strategy she was there to deliver turned out to be piecemeal. It included some numbers on the gender breakdown of staff of the institution but little else. There was no gender assessment of policies and practices of the institution. Her team was just her and one junior colleague. There was no clear workload distribution or allocation system. She had to respond to anything and everything that fell under the general theme of 'gender' or 'women'. This is where the real problems began. Jane had to respond rapidly to every request from the senior leadership, from drafting correspondence, preparing talking points and organising side events to the minutiae of booking hotel rooms for her boss if she was attending an event and was talking about gender and women's health. If the event was linked to gender, she would have to sort it out.

We all have to do things in our jobs that are annoying, and below our pay grade, but can you imagine someone asking a senior male director in a UN agency to do this? Or this happening for any issue unrelated to equality and diversity? Directors are paid to do strategic work, with competing demands on their time as they manage staff, sit in multiple meetings, operate across a range of issues and plot immediate and long-term plans to take an issue forward. Using a director's time on administrative labour that can be done by someone on a lower pay grade is poor management and an indicator that you do not prioritise that person or the work they do. It is also a quick way to devalue both staff and the issue they work on.

The hotel room booking is a part of death by a thousand gender cuts. It is never just one thing if you are the sole gender expert. It is always an accumulation of favours. Everyone is familiar with the sort of day when you get to 5 p.m. and realise you haven't achieved anything on your to-do list because you've been sorting stuff out for other people. This is what it feels like every day to be a gender expert working in a health-related organisation. The favours you have to do. The minutiae of booking things and giving people talking points. Of explaining for the umpteenth time the difference between gender equality and equity, gender lens and gender mainstreaming. Being asked to sit on every panel and in every meeting – except, of course, for the really, really important ones – so that someone can say gender was accounted for. Asking to comment on and review a strategy document, often at the last minute, to ensure gender was included. Responding to last-minute journalist questions. Sitting on countless recruitment panels as you are one of the few women directors (thus ensuring women are represented), despite knowing that the final decision rests with your male boss and if you query this you will be the problem woman. Working in the health sector means you have to adapt your methods to present your insight on gender inequality as a science. When you have to attend an event with your boss (in case there are photos), when you are asked to chair an 'important committee' (that has no budget and which no one listens to) ... The requests even bother you when you're at home, as your phone pings with yet another last-minute WhatsApp favour. You become so used to these requests that you keep your phone by your bed and soon can't sleep as you are accustomed to the disruption. You do it all again the next day. To be a gender expert like Jane you have to be patient as you explain the same point over and over again; you have to be grateful if anyone gives your issue any attention; you have to be across all the other directors' programmes to make the case for why yours matters; and you always have to have one eye on where international politics is headed. You keep going because you know that if you don't do it, no one else will. You do all this as a gender expert motivated by the burning fear that if you don't do it, gender will not be taken seriously and women will lose out.

For Jane, her experience has led her to rethink what she thought was possible to achieve within the UN system. She was fifty-five, had had enough and was getting out. Let the next generation sort it out – although she was clear that she would 'advise young people not to come here'.

Working as a gender expert in a regular health organisation with a low level of interest in gender equality is one thing, but working as a gender expert in health in conflict settings takes this to a new level. Here gender experts are not only responsible for gender-informed policy and strategy, but also act as advocates for the health and well-being of women working in isolated and highly securitised spaces, dominated and shaped by men and masculinity. Being a gender expert in a conflict setting involves helping some of the most vulnerable women and girls in the world, but also internal advocacy to make sure women working in humanitarian and conflict spaces have their health needs met. A gender expert I'll call Linda told me how this double shift works in practice.

Linda's day job in a conflict-affected African country involves stopping the FGM of young girls, preventing child abuse through girls as young as eleven being forced into marriage, and dealing with the huge numbers of fistulas caused by rape and sexual assault. She had been working on women's health issues in conflict and humanitarian crises for years, but experience never made the trauma of her work easier. Neither did being one of the only women living on a military camp away from her family. The only other women on the camp tended to be military, and they only made up 3 per cent of the peacekeepers on base. These camps are so unused to women that when Linda was not dealing with fistulas, FGM and child abuse, she was lobbying on behalf of the women peacekeepers to get the senior command to provide sanitary towels. Meanwhile, women working in a difficult situation just coped with having periods without any sanitary products or had to plan ahead to ensure they had enough to cover their time on mission. Planning may seem simple, but often peacekeepers can be deployed at short notice, and according to the UN, the weight limit of peacekeeper missions is set at 45 kg per person.[2] If you're thinking of your last holiday, where you packed two weeks' worth of clothes, books and sanitary products easily within a 20 kg weight limit, think again. This 45 kg per person rule also includes all equipment – helmets, body armour, weapons. Sanitary products are just one example of the type of lobbying Linda had to do, work that she was not paid or contracted to do, all in addition to a demanding day (and night) job.

Linda also covered the issue of contraception. Given the high-profile sexual assault and exploitation issues perpetrated by UN peacekeepers explored in Part 2, the peacekeeping force takes a zero-tolerance approach to sex. Any peacekeeper found pregnant gets sent home immediately. You are not even allowed to talk about contraception as contraception implies sex. This only goes one way: female contraception is not available and neither are smear tests. However, according to Linda, 'Condoms are very freely available.' As she explained, 'There is no access to any gynaecological care, there is no access to anything related to reproductive health, there is nothing.'

This is how we got on to the subject of self-care for women working in these settings. I wanted to know what her employer was doing to support women like Linda. It is not as if the world does not know the country Linda works in is difficult. There is a deliberate blindness around wanting to open this up, and to think about how to support people who work there. The simple answer is, 'No, it's not available.' As Linda put it to me, 'Sometimes there is like a direct attack in our camp, and of course we are safe, this is not a worry, but you'd think like someone would stop and say "this is really traumatic!" [laughs].'

Linda attributes this in part to the militarised nature of the mission. Attacks happen, you can't make a big deal out of them. However, for the civilian side this is not so easy. As Linda went on to explain:

I just think it's ridiculous, why would you not have space for people to talk about this and then everybody just lectures you 'oh you know you have to self-care' nobody creates the space for self-care it's just crazy. I'm here after some days I'm having nightmares of being bombed and just like yeah, I cannot just walk into a place and say okay let me just have a massage.

Linda was happy to be retiring. The work she did was important to her but she needed to live a life where sanitary products were an essential, not a luxury, and her bosses recognised her mental and physical needs. Where joy was not fleeting. When I spoke to her about the future of women's health, she, like many other gender experts, emphasised her hope for the next generation. Maybe it would be different by the time they came into these roles.

The next generation is something that crops up a lot in conversations with gender experts or women's health activists. It did not escape my attention that the main gender experts I spoke to for this chapter were about to retire or move out of the women's health sector with the hope that the next generation would be listened to. Being the sole gender expert or advocate for women's health is tiring, even more so in conflict and humanitarian settings, so you need youthful energy to carry on pushing for change. I get it. I have taught university students for twenty years, who not only bring new life and perspectives to old topics, but who make me focus on issues I may never have thought of or rethink my own bias. When you get tired of talking about the same inequalities and injustices in the world over and over again, seeing an undergraduate student learn and become impassioned about an issue for the first time – be it the UN engaging in sexual abuse and exploitation, the impact of the global gag rule or the politics of healthwashing – makes you think all is not lost.

The emphasis on young people in global politics is in part the Greta and Malala effect, referring to the global campaigners Greta Thunberg and Malala Yousafzai, who have demonstrated the potential of young women for changing the world. Gender experts in health, and the wider global health community, look at the change, energy and focus these two formidable young women have brought to the issue of girls' education and the climate crisis and imagine the possibilities of a Greta or a Malala for health. She could call out the hypocrisy of governments, demand quicker action on issues of women's health and provide a good source of renewal in thinking about gender and health. Young women bring in new issues and agendas, which can be essential insight and/or correctives for older experts. It is also hard to silence a young person if you are a politician: you don't want to be seen punching down at youthful innocence and energy.

Youth activism to stop FGM is a good example of this. According to WHO figures, over 200 million girls and women in the world have been affected by FGM, with 3 million girls continuing to be at risk every year. In Sierra Leone, the UN estimates that eight out of ten girls (a recent 10 per cent reduction from nine out of ten girls in 2013) have been subject to some form of FGM – either the removal of all or a part of a girl's clitoris (clitoridectomy), and/or the inner labia and/or the labia majora (excision), or narrowing the opening of the vagina by cutting and repositioning the labia (infibulation), or pricking, piercing, burning or scraping a girl's genital area. As you can imagine, after reading the previous sentence, the negative impact on the health of these girls is both immediate and long term. FGM is hugely divisive and taboo as a topic of conversation in, and deeply embedded within the politics of, countries where it is practised. People who have been through the rite of passage associated with FGM don't want to talk about it; people who let their daughter 'go to the bush' don't want to talk about it; other than key activists, those opposed to FGM don't want to talk about it; international donors definitely don't want to talk about it as they don't want to be seen to be getting involved in a country's business; politicians don't want to talk about it unless they are trying to win votes; and as a white European writer I definitely shouldn't be talking about it as I am bringing my Western imperialism to the issue. The people who do talk about it are young women who have been to the bush, run away from the bush, or who want to speak up for those who are not heard.

The amplification of the voices of young women speaking out on FGM is no accident. It is a deliberate political tactic used by activists, international organisations and donors in countries. Many pioneering feminist activists in Sierra Leone are trying to drive change on FGM by introducing alternative rites of passage. They want to maintain the power afforded to women involved in performing these rites – the *soweis*, the most senior women in Bondo society, who are responsible for the rite of passage ending in FGM – *but* get them to stop the final part of the passage: the cutting. While some *soweis* have been supportive of this change, wider uptake has been slow, with those activists pushing for change often dismissed, criticised or labelled as crazy. One way of dealing with this is to switch the spokesperson. If you need someone to speak out about FGM on a public platform who is not going to be attacked or criticised, bring out a young woman to take up the cause. Invest in the creativity and energy of the young, support them with poetry competitions, mural paintings on a public building or funds to run new campaigns. Train them in public speaking and give them a public platform at major events in the country and on the world stage. Make them the future generation of FGM experts. In a society such as Sierra Leone that reveres age, youth can be easily dismissed by politicians and defenders of FGM. However, the international community loves these young people.

One senior gender expert in women's health told me that international donors are always pushing for the new. They want to know who the young feminists are and what they are doing. The effectiveness of young women like Malala, Greta and anti-FGM campaigners is based on how they inspire a wider movement built from the ground up. Young people are central to activist movements as they can bring energy to sustain campaigns on all manner of social justice issues. This is why feminists and gender experts working in women's health often refer to young people as having the potential and strength to take issues forward. But when politicians and institutions begin to take an interest in this activism to advance their own interests and agendas, the vampires come out. The celebration of youth activism can be a means to displace older experts who have become politically inconvenient to politicians or international policy-makers. Young women become the end of the SOS! cycle: first you get a woman leader to deal with the problem and when she's set up to fail, you get a gender expert, and when you don't like what the gender expert or older leader is telling you or they burn out from being asked to explain gender for the 1,981st time, you get the youth on side. You make sure you don't give the youth any real power, and then dismiss them once they are not politically convenient. This is a classic divide-and-rule tactic that diminishes the expertise, knowledge and solidarity of all women in global health.

All the gender experts on women's health I spoke to agreed that three things were essential to success and longevity in the role: 1. good people around you; 2. a good sense of humour; and 3. good data. Part of the problem Jane and Linda faced was that they were on their own: they were the only gender expert in the institution, or were the senior gender person in a small team with a tiny budget. This puts a lot of pressure on individuals to effect change. The experts who faced similar pressures, but had more positive outlooks about the future, all cited tight teams, solidarity or the ability to invest in and look out for the well-being of their team members. The teams they were referring to were either colleagues in their own institutions or the networks and groups they had built up with other gender experts working in different organisations. Informal networks are essential for women working in male-dominated spaces. They are solidarity networks that keep women sane, and in some cases safe. Whisper networks and exchanges are how women circulate information about potential sleazes and predators in their place of work. It was through these networks that women adopted mechanisms such as sitting beside young women new to the WHO so a well-known harasser of women could not be near them.[3] These networks and teams were a space for information exchange, news, gossip and, crucially, laughter at the latest tactics used by colleagues to stop change on gender equality.

Laughter and humour are both survival and strategy in advancing gender equality. There is nothing funny about FGM, maternal mortality or heart disease, but there is plenty to laugh about regarding the absurdity of excuses not to act on these issues. Feminist activists have adopted humour tools such as memes and manel – all-male panel – bingo sheets (filled with excuses as to why there is no woman on the panel).[4] For one of the feminists behind many of these, the activist, artist and academic Saara Särmä, laughter works as a 'common sociality' in that it invites people in to the shared experience.[5]

To understand how humour can work, let me present one of the most common problems people face when trying to advance gender equality in health: gender filibustering. Gender filibustering happens when people do not want to talk about or offer any commitment towards gender equality. Such tactics involve asking for clarification on what key terms such as a gender lens mean, how they apply and why they are relevant. This can go in circles, while the gender advocate has to explain key terms over and over again. The aim is to wear the gender expert down so they give up, lose their temper and in so doing show an unprofessional emotion. Humour is essential to overcoming the gender filibuster: without it you get worn down and think it is an individual experience. It is not.

There are so few gender experts working in women's health that to tell a specific story as to how gender filibustering works in practice risks identifying them and making their work difficult. To protect their identities, and to help you laugh at your own experience or complicity with gender filibustering, I present the Gender Filibuster Bingo Card. Every comment in the square is either directly taken or derived from something a colleague said to a women's health advocate or gender expert in a major international health organisation or to me when I interviewed people in international health organisations (I have heard a lot about men's daughters). The purpose of the card is to tell the story of what women face when trying to advance gender equality in health settings, to build solidarity through laughter and to trivialise the tactics and tiresome ways in which advancing women's health needs is resisted by civil servants, practitioners and people working in health organisations. What is key in the Gender Filibuster Bingo Card is the deflection based on (mis)perceptions of the amount of attention women's health and gender already gets in health policy. It is so absurd and serious, it has to be captured in something as absurd and frivolous as a bingo card to call it out.

To play Gender Filibuster Bingo, check the relevant box every time someone makes one of these comments to you. Once you have a line, you win a small prize of experiencing medium resistance to gender equality in your institutional health setting. And once you've checked all twenty-five squares, you've got the house: you have a fully paid up sexist employer and it is probably time for you to leave.

What about men?	We don't have the budget line.	How are you defining gender?	Member states won't allow it.	Women's health is covered in newborn child mortality.
Where is the data? Is it reliable?	I've done the online gender training.	Do we have a KPI for that?	Everyone is dying.	The problem is that women are poor, not that they are women.
Talk to our gender person.	UNFPA/ UNICEF UNAIDS/ UN Women does women's health, not us.	★ ★ **Gender Filibuster Bingo** ★ ★	I understand the challenges, I have a daughter.	No time for that.
This is an emergency.	Forget about gender, what about race?	Women's health is covered in maternal health.	Not our mandate.	We can't talk about abortion.
You know I'm a feminist.	We need to talk to the youth and see what they think.	Our senior leadership team contains women.	We cover women in vulnerable populations.	Can you do a full gender assessment of our new strategy and get it back to us in a day?

When the laughter runs out you go boring. You reassert existing commitments, you point to the data and you repeat your request and contribution as many times as necessary until someone listens to you. Governments, institutions and employers sign up to all manner of equality laws and agreements. It does not mean they uphold them, but they are supposed to. The tactic of the gender expert is not only to know about these commitments and obligations, but also to build small incremental assurances by the people in charge to ensure that they are paying attention. This builds what is called a path dependency, ensuring that management or leadership follows a specific path on gender equality, that once committed to is hard to divert from. This is boring, repetitive work. But it helps gender advocates hold bosses to account, and depersonalises their own role. They are not the boring gender nag, they are just ensuring that the rules apply to everyone and the institution holds to its own values. The key word in the last sentence is *everyone*; laws and safeguarding practices, for example, must refer not just to senior management or what happens in headquarters, but apply to all behaviour of all staff.

To outsmart the patriarchy it helps to be boring and funny.

You can have a senior woman leading, but she may not represent women's interests. You can have a senior woman shouting for change and trying to get women's issues on the table who is still ignored. You can have all the evidence in the world behind the woman shouting for change, but she will still be seen as a bit too loud and bossy. Fundamentally, all the male allyship, getting women to echo other women, evidence-based practice and adjustments to how you approach the subject is all well and good but, in the end, whether an issue is heard and acted upon depends on whether someone will hear it. And most political systems – whether they be your national government or the WHO – do not think about women's needs, or they do as an afterthought. When it comes to poor women, they both don't think about them and know they don't have to. Gender experts working within these institutions are chipping away at change, building solidarity networks and sharing tips and insights to build the policies that can advance women's health. Not all of them are giving up: lots are in it for the long haul, expecting the backlash, pushing for change.

For women's health and gender experts to be effective, they need laws, policies, targets, strategies, quotas and penalties for when goals on gender equality are not met. There has to be a threat of some kind of loss – financial, reputation, political – to get these agendas on the table. They need humour and networks. These are the tools of any representative and advocate of gender equality.

The final missing ingredient in all of this, the most powerful tool that every gender expert or women's health advocate talks about, is the power of data. Data is the ultimate SOS! As I've shown time and again throughout this book, you cannot get anywhere with stopping women from dying without data.

12

The Power of Data

On 19 March 2020, my phone pinged with a message from a work contact: 'Urgent need for disaggregated data.' Like many people working within governments and international agencies, this senior gender and health specialist was scrambling for whatever information she could find. She knew I had briefed a senior team at the UN on what could happen if the world did not wake up to the impact of COVID-19 on women, and thought I would know where to access good data on this. It was all very well for me to explain what had happened to women in previous health emergencies, such as Ebola and HIV/AIDS, but case studies from previous outbreaks meant very little. Without good current data, senior leaders and governments would not understand how COVID-19 would affect men and women differently and what could be done about it: they wanted numbers of who was getting COVID-19, who was dying from it and who was the most vulnerable.

Data is the number-one currency in the worlds of the UN, foreign aid, health, science and medicine. If you don't have the numbers to show something is happening, then it is not happening. You can have past experience and general trends, but the only language that cuts through is clear numbers: how many people are dying, going to be saved, at risk and can be helped, and how much money it will cost. A consistent theme across the chapters in this book has been the absence of, and need for, better data on how women are dying when they don't have to. Data is the SOS! that will let us know what the problems are with women's health so we can do something about it. This is why when Melinda French Gates talks about closing the gender gap in health, she has pledged $80 million to get better data to do it.[1]

The problem for the person messaging me that morning in March 2020 was that, at the outset of the pandemic, there was no data on gender and COVID-19. Governments either weren't collecting or were not sharing what is called disaggregated data – data that separates issues of incidence (the rate or occurrence of disease), prevalence (proportion of people with COVID-19) and mortality (number of people dying from COVID-19) by gender, socio-economic status or race. Countries share this data with organisations such as the WHO so they can get a global picture of what is happening with an outbreak: where it is coming from and where and who it is spreading to. This is why people go on about track and trace: it is vital to work out the incidence, prevalence and rate of infection to find out what you're dealing with, and track who in a particular population is being infected and dying, to identify both means of transmission and who may be at greater risk so as to protect them.

Not getting good gender data is not unique to COVID-19. It was a full year into the 2014/16 Ebola outbreak before the WHO situation reports disaggregated new infections and deaths by men and women. Non-binary or gender-diverse people did not (and would continue not to) get a look in. After Ebola, some people raised concerns about this, but ultimately the lack of good data on how the emergency was affecting and infecting men and women differently was nowhere in the lessons-learned reports. Good data on gender was an after-thought both during the crisis and when thinking about how to manage future crises better. The same thing happened with COVID-19.

Some countries lack surveillance systems that are able to ac-curately track what is happening in a country. Many countries either cannot or, more likely, do not want to, track how a virus is affecting men and women and/or ethnicities differently. The simple reason offered is many people do not see the virtue of this: viruses don't discriminate in who they infect, so what's the point? Viruses may not discriminate but the societies in which they percolate very much do. The more common ex-planation for a lack of disaggregated data is that countries already have enough on their plates and resist making life more complicated during a crisis. In March 2020, everyone wanted to know how and where COVID-19 was spreading, but no one was thinking about capturing the ways in which COVID-19 was affecting men and women differently. Not collecting the data was a political choice, not a scientific one.

As soon as disaggregated data did start appearing, it shone light on the unequal impacts of COVID-19. It was race not gender that was driving death and disease from the virus. The numbers didn't lie: in some countries people of colour were more likely to die of COVID-19 than white people. The racism was there to see in the numbers. Who lives and who dies is the ultimate barometer of inequality, one which governments do not want people to see.

Data is a device for politicians who do not want to act on an issue. As I explored in Part 2 of this book, the world knows very little about how many pictures of vulnerable children in health settings are available to buy as stock images, how many female health workers are attacked at work, how many women burn out in the health sector. There is a lack of data on these issues because the world does not want to know. If you know, you have to do something about it.

Data is a double bind for women's health advocates. You need the data to prove something is happening. It is an essential SOS! in taking women's health seriously. But no government is going to collect data in the first place unless they think it's an important issue, and they are definitely not going to collect and release data that they don't want you to see. As this chapter will argue, on the one hand data can be an incredibly powerful accountability tool. It gives advocates a clear way of stripping down the rhetoric and lip service paid to women's health, gender equality and racism and getting down to monitoring what is actually going on. In this sense, data is light. It is showing up what is missing and the inequalities and injustices in society that governments would rather you did not see. On the other hand, data can be dark. It can be used to make women invisible, notably women whom politicians want to keep on the margins of society, by either denying their existence or relevance, and by hiding inconvenient health inequalities.

Other than votes, politicians love to bring things down: interest rates, inflation, cost of living, maternal mortality, HIV, cases of COVID-19. One way to pitch an idea to a politician is to give them the data that, if you invest X amount of spending, you can save Y lives. You see these sorts of equations everywhere, from small behind-the-scenes conversations between bureaucrats and strategists when thinking about how to frame an issue, to international pledging conferences where people are trying to get governments to commit funds to specific targets, be it reductions in carbon emissions or reducing child poverty.

A growing trend in women's health is to compare what your money can buy for an issue like maternal mortality in comparison to defence and military spending. For example, at a major UN conference in Kenya in 2019, one speaker, Bruce Rasmussen, calculated $42 billion, or forty-two submarines, was needed to end gender-based violence. Another, Chris Murray, outlined how it would cost $115.5 billion between 2020 and 2030 to scale up efforts to stop 810 women a day dying from childbirth, the exact equivalent of forty-six military planes or 4,277 tanks. This is a clever trick. The military is a costly budget line in government public spending, and the major aid donors – such as the US, UK and France – are some of the biggest spenders on defence. Because military and defence spending is so costly, any comparison shows you get more bang for your buck if you put the money into something else. Compare machines that take life to initiatives that save life, and you have a compelling argument.

Data in this respect is used to attract political attention, funding and commitment. It appeals to politicians, philanthropists and the everyday charity giver: if you invest X you will save Y lives. It is a classic investment model suggesting that if you pay a certain amount in, you will make a substantive return on your investment. You can also track how your investment is doing through quarterly reports tied to clear indicators that measure progress. So not only do you make a commitment to, say, reducing maternal mortality, but you can see where your money is going and what it is doing. The growth in the importance of data, and assessing more bang for your buck in healthcare, has risen alongside the dominance of health and development economics and management consultancy in foreign aid and health strategy and planning.

Since 2000, data has exploded in foreign aid and health metrics, particularly with regard to women's health. As discussed in Part 1, in the early 2000s all UN member states committed to ending poverty by tackling the Millennium Development Goals, three of which were directly related to women's health. A core part of the goals was a set of targets and indicators that would measure progress. Governments would gather data to track this progress and report it to the UN. The UN could then measure what was going well – for example, targets to increase the number of people living with HIV on antiretroviral medicine – and what was not going so well, which was mainly gender equality and maternal mortality. When the MDGs were replaced with seventeen Sustainable Development Goals in 2015, these new goals came with even more indicators and targets for states to be measured against. Aid budgets and funding mechanisms came with their own set of performance indicators, in addition to the global goals they were supposed to align with. This led to an increase in performance metrics in the health and foreign aid sector, and the rise of accountancy firms and data experts to make sense of them. The idea behind the use of such data was twofold. First, measure progress to keep the funds flowing and show what can be achieved if the world put its mind to it. Second, hold governments to account, particularly when they were failing on specific goals, notably those that impacted on women more than men. Use the data to take the politics out of it.

Data, therefore, was a feminist device. It could justify investment in women's health. It could track which governments were doing well on women's health and which weren't. And when governments failed to address women's health, aid agencies would start asking questions and restricting aid flows. Ministers of health could not argue with the numbers (even if they could be selective in how they were used: I'll come to that part).

For gender experts working within the UN, data is not just a bureaucratic tool: it is transformative. Data holds governments and the UN as a whole to account on adhering to their commitments to women's health and gender equality. Data is a means of getting around the diversionary tactics of not talking about gender equality. One gender expert, Lisa, working in the UN, explained to me how the SWAP programme – the not-so-catchy 'UN System Wide Action Plan' accountability framework for gender equality – has moved the institution on ten to fifteen years from where it was on gender issues simply by using data as evidence of where the UN was falling behind. No longer could people ignore the issues or say progress was difficult to measure, because here was the data. For Lisa, the key difference of something like the SWAP was it 'rooted in practice' what gender experts like her had been trying to achieve for years. People wanted to know 'how to' – as in how do you do gender equality, show me how. Such experts would tell colleagues 'this is how you do it' but, more than that, 'this is how we make sure you do it': all through the power of numbers.

Data and numbers are also a way of cutting through the politics. One way of getting people to talk about issues they don't want to talk about is to talk about numbers, not issues. For example, if a government does not want to talk about abortion because it is restricted and does not happen in that country, talk about the PAC numbers instead. PAC numbers refer to post-abortion care (that messy issue from Part 1): civil servants and those working in the health sector know what this acronym means, politicians often don't. Focus on the numbers and acronyms and you avoid the political hot potato. You're just collecting the data on maternal mortality performance. No abortion to see here.

Data is boring. Boring stuff is the perfect way to advance gender equality as few politicians pay attention to detail. If you want to change things, do it through the banal, everyday boring stuff and numbers that politicians like but do not necessarily understand. By making issues banal and boring through the slow burn of the gender experts and bureaucrats we saw in the last chapter, you minimise the political attention.

You can see why data makes such a compelling SOS! It is how you get political commitment, transparency and accountability, and avoid difficult political conversations. The more data and numbers the better. This gives data, and those who work with it, significant power. This power can be positive and transformational in the fight for better health for women. However, this power can also be used to exclude issues, priorities and people. Data, like any form of power, is never without bias. To understand this bias and how data can be used against women, we need to start by thinking about who or what is left out of the data and why. A good way of explaining this is to start with the most difficult challenge: how you collect good data in the first place.

How do you collect data on a virus that no one wants to talk about, in a country with an under-funded and under-staffed health system, and a highly rural population?

In the early years of HIV/AIDS in low-income countries, the answer was to test pregnant women for HIV.[2] Pregnant women undergo blood tests during pregnancy to screen for infectious diseases such a syphilis and hepatitis B that could be harmful to them and their baby. By routinising HIV tests for pregnant women, no one would be singled out or stigmatised for potentially being HIV positive. In some poor and remote locations, getting people into health settings where you can collect the data can be a problem. To get people through the door of a health centre to take the tests and get the data, you have to create incentives. Paying for all men and women to attend is costly, so you concentrate on pregnant women. The payment of small fees or the provision of mother and baby kits to expectant mothers, for example, are a core way of incentivising women to come to clinics regularly throughout their pregnancy, and to give birth in clinics with a skilled birth attendant (a significant factor in reducing maternal mortality).

When getting women to clinics does not work, you send medical teams to the community or train people up within the community themselves (shout out again to the amazing community health workers in Chapter 9). The combination of these initiatives improves maternal mortality, and helps you obtain data. Finally, if all else fails, you can test newborn babies to see if they've been born with HIV. Once you have this data you can then provide a general estimate on prevalence of HIV/AIDS in a given community.

This is how data was generated to estimate the number of people living with HIV/AIDS in low-income countries. In 1998, the UNAIDS/WHO Global AIDS Update reported 29.4 million adults were living with HIV/AIDS around the world, 12.2 million were women, and that women made up 2.1 million of the 5.2 million new cases of HIV.[3] However, this data rested on a particular set of conservative blind spots regarding people's sex lives. First, it assumed that women only have one partner, and that their partner also only has one partner. Second, that men only have sex with women and women only have sex with men. Third, that men and women are equally susceptible to HIV infection. Fourth, that women with HIV attend pregnancy clinics. Fifth, that HIV is only transmissible through sex. And, finally, that women and men are equally able to negotiate safe sex, and have agency over their own health. Those are a lot of big assumptions. When epidemiologists started to dig into this data and refine their methods, and more men came forward to test for HIV, they found that the original data was incorrect. More women were living with HIV than men.

The majority of people living with HIV in the world are women from Southern and Eastern Africa. The drivers are a combination of poverty and patriarchal laws, norms and customs that limit their autonomy over their sexual and reproductive lives, and behavioural factors such as transactional sex, all of which intersect to create cycles of intergenerational risk and inequality. According to the UN's 2022 Global AIDS Update, in 2021 a young woman was infected with HIV every minute. If you were to extrapolate data from women alone, you would both overestimate prevalence rates for the general population and overlook substantive factors that were leading to this difference between men and women. This is a problem that persists in HIV/AIDS data. As one women's health expert put it to me, 'the data dudes are misogynists', as good gender disaggregated data on HIV/AIDS is still hard to come by.

If you are non-binary or gender non-conforming you rarely show up in health data in the majority of countries in the world. When people talk about the 'urgent need for disaggregated data', they are often referring to two genders: male and female. As of 2022, only fifteen countries give legal recognition to non-binary gender in passports, driving licences, birth certificates and other official documentation, with four additional countries having 'some' recognition.[4] Hence, in a world where most countries don't recognise non-binary gender, safe to say few will collate health data for non-binary people, thus erasing them and their needs from the off. This is much the same for trans women. To have targeted HIV interventions for trans women you need data – what risks women face, where they live, how they access health and what they need to live healthy lives. The kicker is most HIV/AIDS agencies rely on data from governments. This depends on governments acknowledging trans women exist in their country. If they don't exist, there is no data; simple maths: $0 = 0$. In a country where there are no trans women, there are definitely no trans women living with HIV/AIDS (or malaria, measles, Ebola, heart disease, a common cold – any health issue really as, remember, they don't exist), so there is no need for a country to do anything about their health needs. In countries where trans women are said not to exist, *and* are marginalised and stigmatised, *and* badly treated by health professionals, they can be completely erased from health data. A toxic combination of denial in the data and poor treatment by medical professionals and health services means in many countries the health needs of trans women are under-resourced and unmet. As Sara M. Davis has shown in her work, NGOs may collate their own data to prove people exist and try to identify such needs, but only government data is recognised as official data.[5] Data can completely erase people's existence. If you erase someone's existence you erase any health needs that may be specific to a part of their identity. Given the power of data in health and foreign aid, this means their needs go completely unseen.

Abortion is, again, another example of how this can work in practice. In Poland, where abortion is illegal in all but a very limited number of cases, but widespread, the government is meant to collect data on the number of illegal abortions that take place. In the past, these abortions were performed by 'the white coat underground' of doctors, but in contemporary Poland, most abortions take place through travel abroad, or are medical abortions with pills supplied by networks of abortion activists.[6] According to leading scholar on the politics of medical abortion, Sydney Calkin, the government is supposed to count the number of illegal abortions to monitor compliance with the law. But the government does not. Or it does and does not release the data. If it did collect the data and made it public it would have to admit the failure of its policy, and how, like in every country in the world, restricting and criminalising abortion does not stop abortion. All governments know this and while some governments aim to punish individual activists, such as Justyna Wydrzyńska, who supplied abortion pills to a woman in an abusive relationship who contacted her for help,[7] few have the political appetite or funds to punish thousands of women. So they just don't count the data, or do and don't release it.

*

The story of HIV/AIDS data points to the importance of disaggregated data and the assumptions we make about the lives of women and men and how similar they are (not). This is the sort of invisible bias that award-winning women's rights campaigner Caroline Criado Perez pointed to in her bestselling book *Invisible Women*. As Criado Perez expertly shows, the world of evidence, data and knowledge is built around men, the male body and the male experience. It is only when a woman points this out or gets hurt that people start to realise it could be a problem. This is mind-blowing when you think of the examples in Criado Perez's book: the absence of women from clinical medical trials and the design of seatbelts and airbags (my own pet peeve: as a woman with big boobs, seatbelts always try to cut me off at the neck). Criado Perez joined a long legacy of feminist philosophers such as Helen Longino, Donna Haraway and Sandra Harding in pointing out that science is not neutral or divorced from the societies in which it works. Decades of evidence of male bias and assumptions about gender roles prove this.

We need good data to correct bias that puts privileged men and their health over that of women. This bias has led to the neglect of a range of health issues that affect women, as there is no evidence or up-to-date data on what is happening to them. More than that, data helps us explain why women are affected by some issues more than men. Some things are physiological. Others are not. HIV/AIDS is a good example of this: more women are living with HIV/AIDS than men because of gender inequality. When we have data that shows this, we can look at what is causing this, point to trends that may shift over time and identify which women are most affected or at risk. We cannot work out why women are dying from preventable causes when we don't have the data on what is killing them and why.

*

Serena Williams knew she was having a pulmonary embolism following the birth of her daughter. As a professional athlete, it was Serena's business to know her health history and understand her body and how to listen to it when something is wrong. She told the nurse. The nurse did not believe her. Serena insisted she needed a CT scan and a blood thinner immediately. The medical team sent her for a CT scan and there they were: blood clots on her lungs. Imagine what would have happened had Serena not been Serena Williams, international tennis superstar, someone whose reputation should mean she commands respect and is listened to? What if she was Serena the accountant, community health worker, lawyer or teacher, a regular African American woman in the US? Chances are Serena would have been another number in the statistics of Black maternal mortality in America.

As Williams wrote about her near-death experience, 'According to the Centers for Disease Control and Prevention, black women in the United States are over three times more likely to die from pregnancy or childbirth-related causes ... this is not just a challenge in the United States. Around the world, thousands of women struggle to give birth in the poorest countries.'[8] In sharing her personal experience, Williams was able to draw attention to one of the most evident and persistent forms of racial injustice in the world: the high rates of maternal mortality of Black women.

In her seminal book *Killing the Black Body*, first published in 1997, Dorothy Roberts systematically broke down how race and racism exploit the bodies of African American women, from the fetishisation and abuse of Black women during slavery to the forced sterilisation of Black women, to the devaluation of Black women's bodies and motherhood. Underpinning all of these issues is the idea that Black women's bodies are somehow 'less': less than white women's bodies and less than male bodies. These are bodies that do not feel pain, or if they do then their pain does not count, and they are not listened to.[9]

In the quarter-century since Roberts's book was published, not much has changed. We may no longer hear about 'welfare queens' in the press, but we do hear about 'strong Black women', a phrase that was once about solidarity and empowerment, but in the medical world seems to be rooted in assumptions around Black women's pain thresholds. Science may have moved on from explicitly talking about eugenics, but when more people of colour were dying of COVID-19 in countries like the US and the UK than white people, leading medical journals such as the *Lancet*, *Health Affairs* and the *Journal of the American Medical Association* still published studies that focused on biological 'difference'. While the work of leading scholars such as Roberts may have brought these racial drivers of health outcomes to the fore, the scientific and health communities will still look for any explanation other than racism.

A common response to evidence of racism in the health sector is that the problems are not really about race at all, but about class and poverty. The poorer you are, the less likely it is that you can afford health insurance and access to healthcare, or make healthier choices such as allocating time for regular exercise and the consumption of healthy foods. The same goes for when you think about the countries with the highest rates of maternal mortality in the world – Chad, South Sudan, Sierra Leone – where the assumption is that these rates of maternal mortality are not because the women are Black, it is because the states in which they live are poor and/or affected by conflict. This overlooks the impact of hundreds of years of the racial capitalism that has contributed to such inequality and poverty. But neither does the argument stack up when you look at Black maternal mortality in a country with a health system where ability to pay does not impact on the healthcare you receive, such as the UK.

A woman giving birth in the NHS should expect an equal service of care to the next woman. Yet, as of 2021, Black women are *four times more likely* to die of pregnancy and childbirth-related complications than white women. That is an improvement from 2019/20, when Black women were five times more likely to die than white women, and Asian women were two times more likely to die than white women. This is not because Asian and Black women's bodies are somehow different from white women's bodies. It is not because Asian and Black women cannot afford to pay for their care. It's about conscious and unconscious racism in the health sector. It does not matter if you are a poor woman in Sierra Leone or international superstar Serena Williams – as a Black woman your pain may be diminished. Your judgement and awareness of your own body may be dismissed. You will still be subject to discrimination and bias.

Data shines a light on this discrimination and bias. It also shows another problem of data. Black women in the UK knew what was happening to them and the women in their lives when they fell pregnant. They were experiencing the pain behind the numbers and talking to people about it. Some researchers were trying to capture the problem but struggled to find research funding to get the data – the currency they needed to be taken seriously. No one believed the experiences of Black women and their families until research was funded on the topic and the first set of results of the MBRRACE-UK study were published in 2018. The results of the study were clear: between 2014 and 2016, white women died from pregnancy and birth-related complications at the rate of 8 per 100,000 live births, whereas Asian women died at the rate of 15 per 100,000 live births, and Black women at 40 per 100,000 live births: hence Asian women were two times more likely to die than white women, and Black women were five times more likely to die than white women.[10]

Since 2020 there has been a substantial increase in public awareness of this issue, in part on account of the advocacy work of groups such as Five X More and The Motherhood Group, prominent Black women working in the health sector such as doctor, activist and author Annabel Sowemimo, and decades of work from leading scholars such as Jenny Douglas. A major turning point was the combination of the unequal impact of COVID-19 on people of colour and the resurgence of Black Lives Matter in 2020, which made the issue of racism in the health sector even harder to ignore. As soon as you had the data, you had the light for activists to use.

The story of Black maternal mortality points to one bigger problem with data on women's health: cis white female able-bodied bias. When I talk about women in this book I mean *all* women: all women's bodies are politicised. If this was to be a continuum, the women whose health is used the most for political ends are those who face intersections of discrimination and inequality, be it women of colour, of low socio-economic status, trans, living with a disability, gay, queer or all of the above. If a male bias exists in science data, there is an additional bias in gender disaggregated data that sees the able-bodied white woman whose gender was assigned female at birth as the norm. These women, women like me, are at the top of the women's health hierarchy.

It is not enough to call for gender disaggregated data about women like me. We need better data to confront the intersecting inequalities that affect women's lives. This is not an impossible or ridiculous thing to ask for. Health leaders and politicians are full of beans as to the potential of smart health and medicine. Smart health and medicine use data and technology to tailor specific interventions to individual health needs. For many in health settings, this sort of smart health-care is the future of medicine: it can be used to predict specific health concerns, understand why your body does or doesn't gain weight, or responds to a certain treatment or virus, and ensure you get the appropriate healthcare for your needs. To say that you can use technology to give me personalised medicine but you can't use technology to collect and analyse data on intersecting inequalities in health is nonsense. If health leaders want to use technology to capture intersecting health inequalities they can. But to do this they will have to demand data to tell them that they should. And for them to get the data, people have to be willing to give it to them.

Whenever my doctor asks if I want to opt in to a more personalised programme of healthcare by sharing more of my health data, I opt out. I live in the UK, so I am not worried about the doctor sharing this information with my health insurance provider and my premium going up. Opting in does not have a material impact on my life. The UK also has clear data protection rules around medical records, so I should be less worried about who this information is shared with. As a professor, I should want my health information to be shared with third-party researchers as that's how health and medicine improve. Opting in is a public good – by opting in not only do I benefit, but so do others. I know – and must strongly re-iterate here – that data protection is taken really seriously by health officials and researchers, and breaches are not only rare but also cause significant sanctions for those in charge. I also know I probably give away far more data and information on my social media feeds than I do to my doctor. But I still opt out. I opt out because I am concerned about the darker side of the growing power and value of data.

When Rosa miscarried after several attempts to get pregnant, the last thing she needed to see was advertising about ovulation trackers on her social media feeds. This was not some cruel twist of fate, or an algorithm that assumed Rosa was a woman of a certain age and therefore the sort of person who wanted to know more about ovulation apps. Rosa had been using an ovulation tracker to follow her periods in order to discover when she was fertile and thus had the best opportunity to get pregnant. The app then had sold her data to Facebook. Facebook knew about her pregnancy loss before she had told her close family. As she put it to me, this advertising was 'obviously quite a triggering thing to do to someone who is experiencing failed pregnancies'.

Two of the biggest period-tracking apps – Flo and Clue – have 46 million and 10 million monthly users respectively. These are regular monthly users; Flo boasts that 230 million women around the world use their app. These apps are part of a huge upsurge of investment in femtech starts-ups. The boom in femtech is directly linked to women's health, and is sold as a means of empowering women to take control of their health through data. In 2021, Flo raised a total of $65 million in investment (just six years after it was founded) and was valued at $800 million.

But then came 2022 and the May leak of the Supreme Court's judgment on the constitutional basis to the right to an abortion in America, ahead of their final ruling on Dobbs vs Jackson Women's Health Organization, which overturned Roe vs Wade. Women's magazines, podcasts and influencers asked the same question in response to the leak, and subsequent Dobbs ruling: should I delete my tracking app to avoid being prosecuted for having an abortion?

The answer in all of these articles and podcasts was yes. Women started deleting their tracking apps.

These apps could track when you were ovulating and when you were not, and when you were pregnant and when you were not. The emphasis being on the not. Data from your phone could be subpoenaed in a criminal case against you to prove you had an abortion. If this data was stored in a cloud owned by a company it could be sold or subpoenaed. This is trickier to do if the data is just held on your own device. But not impossible. Hence, when in doubt: delete.

The doubt was heightened after popular apps such as Flo were controversially found to be selling data to Facebook. This data allowed Facebook to sell targeted advertising; say, buggies to pregnant mums, or ovulation apps to women like Rosa who had just miscarried. Following a *Wall Street Journal* investigation and some backlash against the company, Flo pledged to review and improve its privacy and data practices. After the passing of Dobbs and many women deleting the apps, companies like Flo introduced an 'Anonymous Mode', which allowed customers to use the app without having to input their name or email address. This was done to allow women to track their health 'without fearing for their safety'.[11] Meta, the parent company of Facebook and Instagram, did nothing. It did not even respond to journalist requests for a statement on the matter.[12]

Women were not overreacting. In April 2022, the Norfolk Police Department of Madison County, Nebraska, launched an investigation into the burial of a stillborn baby. A seventeen-year-old girl claimed to have given birth at twenty-three weeks to a stillborn child, and with the help of her mother had buried the body. The police first charged the daughter and mother with 'removing, concealing or abandoning a dead human body'.[13] Two weeks later they introduced additional charges against her mother of providing an abortion as a non-licensed doctor and providing an abortion after twenty weeks. This was the first time in the Madison County attorney's thirty-two years in the job that he had ever brought a charge of this kind.[14] To prove that the seventeen-year-old had had an abortion and that her mum had helped her, the Norfolk Police Department issued a warrant to Facebook seeking data on the mum: her followers, messages on her feed, direct messages between her and her daughter. It was this data that was crucial in bringing the extra charges against the women. In September 2023, the mother was sentenced to two years in prison after pleading guilty to the charges of providing an abortion after twenty weeks, false reporting and tampering with human remains; this judgment followed the daughter's sentence of ninety days in prison and two years' probation for burning and burying a foetus.[15]

Meta insisted that 'much of the reporting about Meta's role ... is plain wrong'. The warrant they received was about the investigation of the 'illegal burning and burial of a stillborn infant'.[16] For anyone with any knowledge of sexual and reproductive rights, this should have raised alarm bells when Meta received it. Even if the bells didn't toll, the wider question of data protection and privacy persists. As Albert Fox Cahn of the Surveillance Technology Oversight Project told the *Guardian*, Meta could have resisted the warrant.[17] They could have launched an expensive court challenge to draw out the process and make it unaffordable for the police department. This may not have changed the outcome of the warrant, but it would have been a warning sign that major tech companies won't roll over in response to data requests.

When the story of Meta's involvement with the Nebraska case came to light in the aftermath of Dobbs, women and politicians became increasingly attuned to how tech companies were handling the data of its users, and how this data could be used to curtail women's sexual and reproductive rights and prosecute women for enacting them. The US Federal Trade Commission published a critical report of Meta's approach to data management, and the US Congress have enacted the My Body, My Data Act to ensure health data is not used to curtail people's rights and bodily autonomy.[18] While welcome, these acts are only catching up. The horse on data regulation has already bolted.

*

Data has been called the new oil on account of the need and demand for it, the wealth it can create and the power asymmetries it can produce. Women's health activists are becoming attuned to the risks of new oil, as well as how hugely valuable to advancing women's health it can be. As data governance and sexual and reproductive rights expert Anja Kovacs put it, current safeguards to protect bodily autonomy are 'completely inadequate'. Data is not something to be mined like a resource, it is something intimately connected to our bodies. Our bodies are translated into data – how much we weigh, walk, eat, sleep – and yet, according to Kovacs, we still lack the language or mechanisms to make sense of this.[19]

We are in deep trouble if we think Silicon Valley is the key to help us make sense of all this. The tech sector makes health look like a feminist paradise. In 2023, only 25 per cent of people working in tech are women, with half of those women leaving the sector before they even reach the mid-career point. Despite initiatives to get more women into tech over the years, this number has held pretty steady. The 25 per cent tend to be located in more 'people'-skilled work if they are white, with women of colour occupying more support/help desk jobs. According to a study from the University of Tennessee (and multiple journalist investigations), the reason women leave the sector is rampant sexual harassment, cultures of misogyny, the severe gender pay gap, normalised abuse and lack of opportunity.[20] And this does not even cover the world of gaming, trolling or TikTok algorithms that promote misogynistic content to young people.[21] Tech CEOs lead the way. Elon Musk, who bought Twitter in 2022 and renamed it X, loves a misogynistic tweet to female politicians, and in 2021 moved his other company Tesla to Texas one month after the state banned abortion.[22] In 2017, Uber CEO Travis Kalanick resigned over sexism in the company; and Meta CEO Mark Zuckerberg admitted to the

US Congress that one of his first initiatives was FaceMash, something he called a 'prank website', which compared the appearance and attractiveness of women. The film *The Social Network* shows FaceMash as the precursor to Facebook, a reference Zuckerberg calls an 'unclear truth'. Genius disrupting trailblazers on gender equality they are not. The new oil of women's health data is owned and controlled by a toxic tech bro culture.

Apps that track your reproductive health were supposed to offer the light of data. We would be empowered by getting to know our bodies more, and holding our womb to account by measuring its performance. However, as with all issues data related, with the light came the dark underbelly of who else could use this data. It could be used not as a means of emancipating women and their health or as an SOS! to unlock the potential of finding out what the real issues are, but as an additional means of controlling women and their health. The problem, yet again, is not the lack of attention to women's health – tech companies, prosecutors and governments are very interested in data on women's health and the power it has – but the wrong kind of attention. This is not attention to advance women's health, but attention to make money from it or, worse, curtail it.

Data is seductive. This is why it is such a compelling SOS! It seduces politicians, policy-makers and gender equality advocates into thinking it is one of the biggest tools we have in identifying and addressing women's health needs. It is incredibly powerful at shining a light on issues, making people take action and holding them to account when they don't. However, there is a dark side to data in how it can be used to erase and obscure some women's very existence and to exploit women and their health even more.

Go back to the start of this chapter, March 2020. Imagine

the change in history if we hadn't had to find the quantitative data to prove what we knew was going to happen to women during a major health emergency such as COVID-19, or listened to Black women when they were seeing friends and family die from pregnancy-related complications. We knew that lockdowns would lead to a rise in intimate-partner violence, that women would shoulder additional burdens of domestic labour and care responsibilities, become the kitchen-table teachers, have to absorb the cost of post-COVID-19 recovery and so on. We knew all of this because we had evidence and experience of it happening to women during the Ebola outbreak, and knew about the burdens women living with HIV face. And yet, because no one built a mega dataset on this past, because there was no political will to do this, there was no 'robust' way of proving it. Imagine what would have happened if we'd asked politicians to prove that this would *not* happen?

The solution to the politics of stopping women dying when they don't have to is not more data and numbers. More data and numbers will just lead to ever more calls for data and numbers until someone is willing to take the data and numbers seriously. Women's lives do not need to be costed in comparison to fighter jets and tanks, or presented as an investment portfolio that will generate a specific societal return. The solution is much simpler: it is about believing women.

The way we stop women's exploitation, the rolling out of SOS! – demands for more women leaders, more data – and the politicisation of women's health is simply to believe women. Believe women when we are in pain. Believe women when we are attacked for the work we do. Believe women when we say we know what is best for our health. Believe women when we tell you our body is a woman's body. Believe women when we show you our qualifications and experience. Believe women when we fear public health measures such as lockdowns and quarantines are a threat to our safety and well-being. And believe women when we say politicians are trying to kill us.

It is when we believe women that we stop the sick politics of women dying when they don't have to.

Conclusion

The Driver and the Green Wave

The pink house on the corner of Fondren Place and North State Street is unapologetic. Sitting across from a hotel, a taco shop, a chicken and burger joint and a thrift store in the Fondren district of Jackson, Mississippi, you cannot look away from it. The main front entrance is all boarded up and the side entrance is covered with beige tarpaulin with a temporary entrance cut into the middle of it. The only disturbance to the pink house with the mint roof is contractors parking their trucks at the back next to the giant lime-green skip, rigging the occasional ladder and generally mooching around the building. Dotted among the black railings is the occasional yellow 'No Trespassing' sign. According to the Jackson rumour mill, the plan is to turn the pink building into retail shops.

The only sign of what this house once was is the three white stone carvings above the main entrance. The central stone carving is a woman with wings flanked by a woman holding a child and a man looking on. This is a building of solidarity, community, prioritising and believing women. The pink house was once the home of Jackson Women's Health Organization, the only abortion provider in the whole of the state of Mississippi. Looking at it in November 2022 you wouldn't think that this building is the epicentre of a ruling that changed the world.

The pink house was at the heart of the US Supreme Court's 2022 ruling Dobbs vs Jackson Women's Health Organization et al., the ruling that said the US constitution does not protect the right to abortion, and which ended one of the most fundamental sexual and reproductive rights for Americans. Dobbs overturned Roe vs Wade, the 1973 Supreme Court ruling that protected the right to an abortion based on the constitutional right to privacy rather than the right to equal protection before the law. The Dobbs ruling made abortion up to the discretion of individual states in the US. Passed on 24 June 2022, the ruling sent ripples of disbelief, fear, jubilation, emboldening and gut-wrenching sickness across the world. Abortions became illegal overnight in the states of Alabama, Arkansas, Idaho, Kentucky, Louisiana, Mississippi, Missouri, Oklahoma, South Dakota, Tennessee and Texas. The US had crossed to the other side and was on a path followed by many other countries in the world, curtailing one of the most important forms of healthcare for women. America followed other countries such as El Salvador, Honduras and the Dominican Republic in tightening limits on abortion, marking the 2020s as a period in which women's reproductive rights and freedoms were getting seriously worse.

Before the ruling in June 2022, there was no peace for the pink house. As the only place you could get an abortion in the whole of Mississippi, it was busy with people seeking abortions and other people trying to stop them entering. The pink house was already subject to scrutiny, having been the centre of the initial case against Thomas E. Dobbs of the Mississippi State Department of Health after state law banned abortion after fifteen weeks of pregnancy in 2018. The house was constantly surrounded by anti-abortion protestors holding up posters of foetuses, signs saying 'Murderer', and bullhorns. When they weren't standing outside the pink house they were trying to disrupt LGBTQ+ pride events.

Their main target was the (mostly) women and pregnant people wanting to enter the house. These women were protected by defenders. Defenders are mainly women, in this case predominantly women of colour, who are activists steeped in reproductive justice and organising to support women's access to healthcare and reproductive choice. They are not about stopping women having children: far from it, they are about giving women choice over their reproductive lives to have as many or as few children as they want. They not only protect the women entering the building from protestors, they also play a pivotal role in educating people working in the sector that abortion is about more than health, it is about justice.

Four months after the ruling, the protestors had gone. The owner of the clinic had packed up and moved on to New Mexico. Journalists had filed their stories and were focused on the 2022 mid-term elections. Abortion was a key election issue, but the centre of gravity had shifted from a fleeting moment in the American South back to the usual political hubs of the northeast. Other than the pink house itself, decorated with tarpaulin and builders' ladders, there was little to suggest that this Jackson street had once been the centre of debate over women's bodies around the world. It was over.

But it was not over for women needing abortions.

Three times a week, sometimes more, the driver drives the 1,200-mile round trip to one of three abortion clinics in Illinois. Her passengers are always strangers. She doesn't need to know their names, and it's best that she doesn't. The less she knows about them, the more she can protect them from law enforcement. The journey takes roughly eight to nine hours one way depending on traffic and the need to stop.

When you are driving pregnant women, you take a lot of stops to pee, to snack and to pee again.

You never talk about why a woman needs an abortion. People need abortions for all manner of reasons, some of which can be deeply personal. This can be the simplest: they got pregnant by accident, didn't realise they were pregnant and didn't want to be, changed their mind or their circumstances changed. Or the more complex: the need for an abortion is related to violence and abuse; for example, a woman's pregnancy is the result of rape, or because a relationship has broken down. Then there are the health issues (which can also intersect with the above): the pregnant person's life would be at risk if they continued the pregnancy, or their mental health would suffer, or the foetus has shown abnormalities that would minimise the chance of any newborn child surviving. And then there are the needs that policy-makers deliberately forget, that medical and surgical abortion procedures can be necessary to manage pregnancy loss. Pregnancy loss is extremely common, with an estimated 23 million miscarriages in the world every year, and is still not spoken about openly, with many people having to deal individually and privately with their loss.[1] Stigma and legal restrictions around abortion can compound the isolation around pregnancy loss, but do not stop women needing medical and surgical help. For as long as people can get pregnant, there will be demand or need for abortion. And for as long as activists provide abortions, they'll never ask why. There is no hierarchy to why someone wants an abortion in the world of reproductive justice.

If you have funds and control of those funds you can book a few days' holiday and fly to another state to get an abortion. This is not simple and involves time and organisation – not just flight, hotel and abortion booking, but time off work, and organising childcare if you have other children. There is also the emotional cost – both of having to go through all this and of having to explain why you're travelling out of state for three days. But it is doable. For people who do not have funds, or control of their money, getting an abortion may seem impossible, unless they are plugged into the networks. They rely on women like the driver.

The clinics in Illinois serve people from Mississippi, Texas, Alabama and Louisiana. Sometimes there are more women than there are people to help them. When the clinics were oversubscribed during the first year after the ban, the activists put women on a plane to Florida, until Florida became uncertain. In 2022–3 Florida was still an option, but then politicians began to pass legislation to propose a fifteen- and then a six-week limit on abortion. It cost on average $2,000 per person to send someone to Florida, taking into account flight cost, hotel, ground transfers, food and drink and the abortion itself. And that was just the financial cost. Then there were the additional risks. Many of these people had never left the state of Mississippi or been on a plane before. If you've travelled on planes within the US you know that delays and cancellations are part of the process. They are a massive inconvenience and can be costly. For a frequent flyer, the best thing to do is shrug it off and flex your credit card for some sleep and snacks and claim on insurance later. This was not a luxury women flying from Mississippi to Florida could afford. Activists like the driver dreaded the holiday season, when flight costs would shoot up, get over booked, and airports – not always the friendliest of spaces at the best of times – would become even more hectic. The driver feared people in need missing connecting planes, being stranded with no money, still pregnant, on their own as they tried to get across the country for an abortion.

On the days the driver is not behind the wheel, she is organising. Her phone is constantly ringing and pinging – I lost count of the number of times it went off during the hour and a half I spent with her in a Jackson coffee shop. When her phone was not pinging, she would be looking around the room, scanning it for anyone who was coming in, or listening to our conversation. It is not just the driving and phone messages: reproductive justice work in the Deep South of the US is one of being in a state of constant vigilance.

In mid-2023, driving someone across state lines to get an abortion was not illegal in Mississippi. But the change was coming. In April 2023, Idaho was the first state in the US to pass a law that criminalises any person who helps someone get an abortion, medical or surgical. One of the most common forms of abortion is medical abortion – the taking of two pills: mifepristone and misoprostol. Mifepristone has been approved for use by the US Food and Drug Administration (FDA) since 2000, and while misoprostol is approved for other medical uses, it has not been approved for abortion in the US. In January 2023, the federal government, the FDA, eased restrictions on how women could access medical abortion by allowing the pills to be over-the-counter in pharmacies. This would help women access medical abortion, and give activists another line in helping women, by moving pills instead of people across state borders. However, states that banned abortion were already hip to this. In a state like Idaho, anyone providing abortion pills or driving someone across state lines to an abortion clinic could face two to five years in prison. Oklahoma and Texas were yet to pass similar laws, but did permit lawsuits to be brought against people like the driver. And at the time of writing, the US Supreme Court was tying itself in knots over whether to change FDA rules and restrict access to Mifepristone.

Activists knew that politicians would stop at nothing to restrict the sale of abortion pills, and to prosecute women seeking them and those who provided them. They were constantly vigilant. They were relying on some of the most effective SOS! that have saved women for years: networks, local direct action and connection to a movement that was bigger than Jackson.

Driving strangers 1,200 miles, three times a week, at risk to her own safety, freedom and well-being, is non-negotiable for the driver. She has to do this work. Drivers like her are doing it for *all* women and people in need of abortions. All the SOS! of more women leaders, gender experts and better data on the danger of unsafe abortion adds up to very little for the driver. The driver knows the threat is real, that the abortion ban was coming. She is well aware that the politicians coming for women's right to healthcare often cut their teeth on curbing the rights and lives of the most racialised and marginalised women, notably trans women. For the driver, there is only one SOS! – the conviction that if she doesn't act, women will die. She is not responsible for the law but feels responsibility for the women she drives; for all women, for that matter.

There was a saying that a number of Jackson women repeated to me: 'No one is coming to save us.' No one was looking to the South before, and no one was looking now. Ever since the non-consensual sterilisation of African American women got so common that it became known as the 'Mississippi appendectomy', activists and regular Mississippians have been aware of how state politicians can and will exploit and control women's health as a political tool. Years before the passing of Dobbs, activists in the South had been warning that the threat to women's lives and reproductive rights had never gone away. The passing of laws in other Southern states, such as the 2021 Texas SB8 banning abortion after six weeks of pregnancy (a time period when most women often don't even know they are pregnant), was a sign of things to come.

Mississippi has some of the worst outcomes of maternal, newborn and infant child mortality in America. The state

guidelines are clear that sex education must focus only on abstinence or abstinence plus, stressing abstinence but including
information on contraception. When the federal government
offered to give the state money to extend Medicaid to women
up to twelve months post-partum – a core intervention to
improve the health of new mothers and babies – the state
at first rejected it. The rejection had nothing to do with the
health of the mothers and babies – it was about politics.
Mississippi was one of ten Republican states wanting to resist
any expansion of Medicaid – a core part of the Affordable
Care Act, aka Obamacare, Democrat President Barack
Obama's flagship attempt to make healthcare affordable to
all Americans. Resistance to the extension of Medicaid in a
poor state like Mississippi led to a hospital crisis as costs spi-
ralled, but the state legislature still refused to accept money
from the federal government. One report from the Office of
the State Economist of Mississippi estimated that accepting
the extension would release $1.35 billion in federal funds to
healthcare, which would be of massive help to hospitals struggling with demand.[2] Only when the situation with Medicaid
became politically contentious did the state of Mississippi
relent and extend its cover to women and their babies twelve
months post-partum. Saving mothers, again, was good politics. Everyone else, not so much. That's how bad it is for new
parents: you've got some of the highest risk to your health and
well-being, the federal government wants to help, but still the
state says no until it is better politics for them to relent.

Finally, sterilisation still happens, but the type of women
this now affects has changed, shifting from African American
women to undocumented migrants. Still women of colour,
but predominantly from Central and South America. While
already suspected in some states, the issue came to light when
Dawn Wooten, a nurse who worked at an ICE (Immigration
and Customs Enforcement) detention centre in the Southern

state of Georgia, blew the whistle on a high number of hyster-
ectomies of migrant women, calling one male gynaecologist
'the uterus collector'.[3] Despite threats and intimidation,
forty women have since submitted a case against the state of
Georgia based on what the uterus collector did to them.[4]

Before Dobbs, women in Mississippi knew how attacks on
women's health unfolded and were working within the communities they lived in to improve women's health. Community
activists and health workers told women what their choices
and rights were, how to access reproductive health services
for free, what services to expect and demand. They mon-
itored those services to ensure they had the right training
to inform women of *all* of their options, and worked with
teenagers and young people to talk about their own sexuality, and with their parents and grandparents, who had been
shut off from access to information because of the Jim Crow
laws that racially segregated US Southern states and limited
their access to education. They tried to capture federal funds
to take women's health out of political institutions and into
non-profits. Mississippi may have some of the highest rates of
teenage pregnancy and economic poverty, and that shapes a
great deal of people's lives, but it is balanced by the high levels
of organisation and activism from Mississippians in trying to
change this. Mississippi women were not waiting and looking
for outside help as they knew to do so would mean waiting
for ever.

The very real fear is that the Dobbs ruling will kill women
in these states, push many into poverty, or even worse poverty,
criminalise them and cause incredible harm and pain. The
rest of the world started to notice this threat only when it was
no longer just happening to women in states like Mississippi.
The uncomfortable truth of people turning a blind eye until
it happens to them has been consistent in this book, whether
I am talking about HIV/AIDS, Ebola, healthcare workers

or COVID-19. The problem has never been a lack of data, women leaders or someone raising the flag for attention: from abortion in Mississippi to Ebola in Sierra Leone, women have been signalling the problem and acting on it. Women's health is always under threat and women are always picking up the pieces of bad politics that cause harm and death. One thing that unifies so many stories in this book is that it has consistently been Black women who have been ringing the warning bell as to how politics is affecting their health and well-being, and taking direct action themselves. Women know they cannot rely on the SOS! being proposed by policy-makers – more women leaders, more gender experts, better data – that have not served them in the past. So instead they depend on some of the oldest and most effective solutions: taking direct action, building networks and a movement.

The driver told me she is following the path of many women and activists who have helped save lives, from Harriet Tubman, one of the 'conductors' of the Underground Railroad (the network of safe transportation and accommodation that helped those who had escaped their enslavement), to those who helped Jewish people escape the Nazis. The driver is another link in the history of underground abortion networks, such as the white coat underground in Poland, or the Jane Collective in Chicago, set up in 1969 to help women seeking abortion until the passing of Roe vs Wade in 1973.

Such networks are fundamental for women accessing healthcare around the world, picking up the gaps that the international community forgets. In the first year following the 2022 Russian invasion of Ukraine, 8.1 million people left the country, the majority of whom ended up in Poland. Ninety per cent of the people who made up this mass migration were women.[5] Some of these women found themselves pregnant – some as the result of rape by soldiers – in a country that prohibits abortion. When faced with the trauma of flee-ing their country and an unwanted pregnancy, it was again women's networks and groups that stepped in to provide advice and access in Ukrainian to the underground network in Poland.

Across the world these networks prevent unsafe abortion and the unnecessary death of women by sourcing and posting abortion pills, and offering phone consultations and online guidance on how to have a medical abortion. They fly drones into countries to drop off abortion pills, recommend travel companies that specialise in accessing abortion across state or national borders and, of course, drive women to clinics. There is a whole infrastructure providing women with the healthcare they need when governments try to stop them.

Networks depend on quiet whispers to keep the women they help safe. But there is a limit to quiet whispers. To ad-vance change you need to be loud about abortion, to break the stigma and show it is an everyday occurrence in the world, not limited to survivors of rape or violence but a procedure women you know have had for a variety of reasons. Latin American feminists have pioneered the method of speaking openly about abortion, calling it 'social decriminalisation' – if the law doesn't follow, at least change the minds of society.[6]

Women on Waves, a collective of activists led by Dutch doctor, Rebecca Gomperts, is a good example of normalis-ing abortion. Women on Waves provide abortions in a fully equipped shipping container, twelve miles from the shore of countries that have abortion bans, where waters become inter-national and thus not subject to national abortion laws. The ship does not arrive in ports quietly under the cover of night. It does so proudly in full daylight, with the hotline number for women to call displayed on its side. This is both to get the word out to women who want an abortion and to use the boat as a platform to bring attention to abortion and normalise it.

Often the ship is met with protest. In 2004, the Portuguese government sent a warship to stop the Women on Waves boat from docking in the port. The warship sailed right into the activists' trap: they got more attention for the cause and took the Portuguese government to the European Court of Human Rights and won. The boat was a deliberate provocation. The boat has now shifted more to the online supply of medical abortion pills through Women on Web, but founder Gomperts still engages in high-profile actions to raise awareness of how common and necessary abortion is as a basic right. This is what change in abortion law depends on – how you change the minds of people in society and create an awareness of how common and everyday abortion is. The connection with women you know is what made activism in countries such as Ireland and Colombia so effective. The same applies to all of women's health. You fight for change in law and through political pressure, but change comes from everyone realising the everyday harms being done to women in their lives.

In the early hours of Wednesday 30 December 2020, a sea of people waving green flags anxiously waited outside Argentina's Congress in Buenos Aires. Vast crowds don't usually come together in their masses to watch livestreamed debate in the government's second chamber. After twelve hours watching a contentious debate, a collective scream of celebration emanated from the green sea and the anxiety dissipated into joy, as the crowd realised they had won. Following decades of grassroots campaigning, mobilising celebrities behind their cause and political activism within government, the green wave had crashed: abortion was legal in Argentina. Like Ireland before it, Argentina showed it was possible to change abortion laws in Catholic countries by forming a movement, in this case *la marea verde*, the green wave.

If anything symbolises effective leadership and a pathway

to change women's health it is not any charismatic individual: it is the colour green. Green was chosen by abortion activists in Argentina to represent nature and life on the planet, to deliberately reclaim discussions on life from the 'pro-life' movement. It was meant to normalise the everyday presence of abortion in women's lives and to be inclusive of everyone in the gender equality movement.

Who used something first is always contested, but the idea for a unifying visual identity drew on the political legacies of female activism in Argentina, most notably *Las Abuelas y Madres de Plaza de Mayo*/The Grandmothers and Mothers of the Plaza de Mayo. The peaceful protest of *las Madres*/ the Mothers against the military junta that ruled Argentina between 1976 and 1983 has taken on almost folkloric significance in women's activism and peace studies. In 1977, a group of Mothers and Grandmothers went to one of the main squares of Buenos Aires, the Plaza de Mayo, wearing white cloth nappies on their heads as headscarves, clutching pictures of their 'disappeared' children. They would stand in front of the pink government building (pink because opposition parties would take it in turns to paint it alternatively red and white depending on who was in power), often in silent protest, a reminder to the ruling military junta that they knew who was responsible for the disappearance of their children, and they would not let them forget it. When the Mothers first started to gather in the square in 1977, Argentina's rulers didn't know what to do with them. They were Mothers and Grandmothers, the symbol of life, birth and maternal love, the future of Argentina: you could not just attack Mothers. The Mothers knew this, using their status and the white nappy scarves as a symbol of peace. Eventually security forces expelled the Mothers from the square, but they kept up their protest, refusing to be silenced, refusing to be moved. Even when one of the founding Mothers, Azucena Villaflor, was disappeared, they persisted. The powerful image of Mothers and Grandmothers standing up to fearsome military rule gave hope to many Argentinians and spread throughout the world as a symbol of women's resistance to state terror. Even today, some of the Grandmothers and Mothers who are still alive meet every Thursday in the square. They continue to campaign until every disappeared person is accounted for, and every child taken by the junta is united with their family. Every time the Mothers find another missing child and reunite them with their family, the country celebrates.

In 2015, the women's movement once again wanted politicians to watch Argentina, and again they used a colour for their protest, this time green. Protestors took to the streets and social media to ensure not one more woman, or #NiUnaMenos, would suffer at the hands of gender-based violence. At the time, gender-based violence in Argentina was at a rate of one murder every thirty-five hours.[7] For the women's movement, this constituted a femicide: women were dying because of misogyny and patriarchal politics. Grassroots movements started to wear *pañuelos verdes* – green scarves. Teenagers started to wear them on their school backpacks. The green scarf became a symbol of everyday resistance and solidarity. You could try to kill women, silence women, stigmatise them, but they would wear the green scarf as a sign that they would not be stopped, and more than that, they had had enough: not one more woman would be killed by gender-based violence.

Abortion was always a part of the movement. Restriction of abortion rights as an act of misogyny, political power over women and, for some, a wider part of violence against women, meant that rapidly the symbol of the green scarf became about more than violence against women: it was a national symbol of all the issues that harmed women and their fight for equality, including abortion. By 2018, in the build-up to the first vote on abortion laws in the country, the green scarf was so popular in Argentina and so ubiquitous at rallies, on backpacks and wrists of women that the country ran out of green fabric. The bill did not pass in 2018, but a movement and symbol of resistance had been born, spreading across Latin America and creating the *marea verde*: the green wave, culminating in the 2020 change. Women in Chile, Colombia and Brazil adopted green scarves with their own slogans (e.g. *causa justa* – just cause – in Colombia) as a means of putting pressure on their own governments and building a movement across borders.

The movement built on decades of activism across borders and the work of women like the driver. For the movement, women's health was never distinct from gender inequality, but a fundamental part of it. The green wave always understood women would never be free to live their lives as long as the state could take away a basic right to health. While abortion galvanises the movement and gets attention in the news, the commitment to women and their health is always about bodily autonomy, and the freedom for women to live and not die when they don't have to. It is about calling out the politics of what makes us sick. As this book has shown, abortion is just one part of this. The politics go much deeper. The green wave is about stopping the sick politics of women dying for another person, country or institution's political gain.

When the US Supreme Court voted in favour of Dobbs, New York congresswoman Alexandria Ocasio-Cortez tossed a green scarf over her shoulder as she spoke to activists about the need to mobilise. She followed in the footsteps of Representative Nydia M. Velázquez from New York, who had prominently worn her green scarf to the Capitol.[8] In Argentina, the green movement gathered outside the US embassy in solidarity with American women. Green is a symbol of the SOS! that works, a network and movement between women across the world who believe that change does not come from one woman, one country, or rich, white women, but from building solidarity.

What happened in Mississippi is part of a global sickness of women dying when they don't have to because of politics, and then women trying to stop this from happening, pushing back and dealing with the consequences. It does not matter if you live in one of the poorest countries in the world, like Sierra Leone, or the richest, America: this sick politics is global. This is not a passive politics, it is one of actions and decisions taken (predominantly by men) and then dealt with and resisted by women in order to keep women alive. We can see it, we know how it affects our lives and kills women, how women's health is always a proxy for something else, and we are sick of it. We know how to stop women dying when we don't have to; the evidence of what works is there and we have the pledges from governments around the world. The problem is a sick politics that exploits women, does not believe women and stigmatises women. To break this politics, you need the most effective form of SOS! – direct action, networks and movements that don't wait for someone to come and save us, or accept piecemeal funding or concessions with the promise of future change, and is constantly vigilant to attacks on all women's health. We ignore networks, health professionals and activists and their warnings about women's health at our peril.

The activists driving 1,200 miles three times a week told me.

The women's health experts trying to protect women in Ebola quarantines in Sierra Leone told me.

The women working to try and get their colleagues in the UN to take women's health seriously told me.

The nurses at the front line of patient frustration and violence told me.

The community health workers who are always asked to step up in an emergency but were never paid told me.

And the public health workers facing another round of austerity cuts to their budgets told me.

It is time we believed them.

Until then the drivers will continue to take to their cars and transport anonymous women thousands of miles, stopping for pee and snack breaks. And then they do it all over again. To keep women alive.

Epilogue

What Next?

I teach international politics to undergraduate and postgraduate students. At the start of every academic year I conduct a range of ice-breakers to get to know students. Students can often be quite shy at the beginning so I always ask the easy, standard question: why did you decide to study international politics? Some students say they enjoyed studying the topic at school or college, quite a few have interesting life stories that they want to make sense of, and others say they thought politics seemed more interesting than the law degree their parents wanted them to do. Every year a high number of students are motivated to study politics because they see inequality and injustice in the world and they want to do something about it. Their desire and energy to change the world does not shift over the course of their degree. If anything, the more they learn, the more it grows. What does start to creep in is a helplessness about the scale of inequality and injustice being all too big, too complex and too much to take on. The more they know, the more they feel the world is impossible to change.

Chances are you have finished this book and may be feeling like my students: angry at the world and motivated to do something, but at a loss as to what that could be. Maybe you want to travel to Mississippi, buy a car and drive women across state borders to get an abortion, but then remember you are down to do the school run tomorrow. Perhaps you have spent years giving to charitable organisations such as MSF, and are now confused as to whether you should stop your monthly donation. Maybe you have worked for some of the organisations and governments in this book, feel deeply loyal but oddly conflicted as you have tried to change things, but kept coming up against brick walls, got worn down and had to step back for your own sanity.

Feeling helpless gets us nowhere. There are no quick-fix solutions to the issues in this book, but there is always something you can do. All of us are restricted by time, money, age, ability, the type of jobs we do, race, gender, security, discrimination, where we live and so on, so there is no one size fits all to how to do something, and plenty of reasons for us to not do anything. The trick is to think about what you want to do and are able to do. For example, I was once at an outside conference by the gates of an international arms trade fair in London. While listening to a speaker talk about the ethics of violence to very interested academics and mostly bemused commuters, a lorry with a major rig on the back pulled up in front of us. Within seconds, anti-arms-trade activists clocked that the load was a tank and lay down in front of the lorry to stop it entering the trade fair. I froze, not knowing what to do. I was willing to lie down but was waiting for someone to tell me to. And, if I'm honest, I was worried that I didn't know how to lock on, and what if I was arrested? I realised in that moment that I am a rubbish direct-action kind of person. But just because I didn't lie down in front of that tank doesn't mean I can't use my skills in other productive ways. Same for you.

So, what can you do next? To make this as user friendly as

possible, I've divided suggestions into two sections – The Easy Stuff and Worth the Effort. You can pick and choose across the sections, and come back to different options over the years as your circumstances, finances, expertise and commitments change. You may never face discrimination at work, or come across a case of exploitation and abuse, and hopefully you never will, but if you do you can come back to this resource years from now to help you. You know how you move in the world, how people see you, and the structural barriers you're up against every day so what I suggest may be totally unhelpful to your situation right now. Changing the world to improve women's health is much like the perennial how do you eat an elephant question (I mean first, why would you want to?): one spoonful at a time.

The Easy Stuff

1. Do nothing

First, do absolutely nothing if you don't want to. Reading this book and understanding how politics in the world leads to women dying when they don't have to is already a lot. Once you understand something you can see it for what it is and start recognising patterns. You can call these out, or not. But understanding the situation and what is going on gives you power.

Women are often made to feel responsible for fixing problems in the world, and this book has shown that this can lead to their exploitation, particularly in the world of health. I want to live in a world where women are left alone to live their lives, and can become active in certain issues if they want to, not because someone is telling them to or making them feel guilty. Same if you're a man or non-binary. There's all the being an ally stuff which is great – and I've added some ways you can do this below – but sometimes it would be good if men specifically did nothing. Part of the problem is men's exploitation of women's health for political gain. The aim therefore is inaction – stop exploiting women's health – not action.

Doing nothing may feel tricky. Think about the gender experts in Chapter 11 or the health professionals in Part 2 who took on more and more work, regardless of the risk to their own well-being. No one person can do everything on their own. Social media and tattoo slogans and quotes (seriously, I once met someone with a tattoo of one of the following quotes) such as 'silence = complicity/violence', 'Be the change you want to see in the world', or 'The only thing necessary for evil to triumph is for good men to do nothing' are not necessarily wrong, but should not be a guide to life and definitely not make you feel guilty for inaction. Guilt over inaction is a powerful way for people to exploit you. Don't let them.

Do nothing so as to do no harm. You may be uncomfortable about some of the topics raised in this book. For example, you may understand that abortion bans don't stop abortion and can actually harm women, but your faith or values makes you uncomfortable about abortion. You may feel conflicted, or less confident talking about women's health in war. In these situations, do nothing. No one is asking you to give money, advocate or volunteer for something that makes you feel uncomfortable. But likewise, don't spread misinformation, vote for people wanting to curtail women's health or be complicit in the harm of other women. If you don't want to actively call something out, at the very least don't defend the exploitation of women's health: do nothing.

2. Play bingo

Use the bingo card in Chapter 11. Share it with your friends and colleagues. This will help you entertain yourself and look attentive in online meetings (use at your own risk during in-person meetings), and will make you and others feel less alone when you are listening to another filibuster against change. Develop your own bingo card to fit with your own needs.

3. Become a dog

The bingo card also relates to another tip: become a dog. Dogwhistling is when politicians use coded words that say one thing, for example, 'inner city crime', that means something else – 'black people in cities commit all the crime' – for their core base of supporters. As the example I used demonstrates, dogwhistling is often used to mask derogatory, offensive or discriminatory views. Other examples are the use of 'global elite' or 'international banks' as code for the anti-Semitic sentiment that money and banking are controlled by Jewish people; or 'Real Americans', meaning white Americans who were born in the USA – a way for politicians to appeal to white supremacists without going the whole hog and popping on a white hood. There are a range of dogwhistle terms that refer to women's health – family values or traditional values, gender ideology, matters of conscience – each of which refers to curtailing women's sexual and reproductive rights. Politicians use these phrases to test the water with their supporters. The trick for you is to be attentive to such words and phrases, and as soon as you hear them – if you wish, this is the easy action section, after all – get mobilised. Get mobilised means call them out, contrast their views with the existing laws and protections on women's health. Identify where they are seeking power and join networks to campaign to keep them out of power. Finally, identify their political networks and where they are getting funding from: this is how you can point to growing trends locally, in other parts of your country or the world.

4. Spend your vote and your money wisely

Where you spend your money has power. Don't buy from companies that fund politicians and organisations that seek to curtail women's health. This may take ten minutes of your time, probably more when you go down the political funding rabbit hole. First, identify politicians who vote against key efforts to stop women dying when they don't have to – those who stop FGM bans, introduce abortion limits, curtail budgets on maternal mortality, disinvest from breast cancer, and so on. Don't vote for them. Second, look at who contributes to their political campaigns. Third, don't buy anything from these companies, or from the individuals who derive their wealth from these companies and donate to political campaigns. Sometimes you might use these companies when you're short on time or need the convenience they offer. Don't be hard on yourself about this or let it derail your efforts. No one is perfect.

5. Don't get stuck in feedback loops (that go nowhere)

Never advocate for woman's health as a means to something else. For example, don't fall for the argument that if you invest money in keeping women alive and healthy they will bring thousands of dollars into your economy; or you need to support women during a health emergency as they're the ones who will relay messages home and keep the family in line with lockdowns and quarantines; or get women to be leaders in your health organisation as they will then represent every issue on gender equality you can think of. Making a case for women's health or justifying an investment in women's health should only and always be about women's health needs. Nothing else. If you accept something is good for women, that should be enough.

'But that's not how the world works!' I hear you cry. True, the 'invest in women, invest in the world' mantra is everywhere and hard to beat, and this is how the world works. But as this book has shown, this mantra is getting us nowhere. We've made the investment case for women's health for decades and yet ... If you make women's health about something else, then you enter a constant feedback loop of having to assert all the added benefits to wider society of doing something for women, rather than just focusing on the fact that it would be good for women. If this is how the world works, the world is not working for women.

This applies to more than women's health. It applies to every woman's issue or woman advocating for what she wants.

6. Take care in what you share

Remember how experts call data the new oil? Information about your health and body is a mini oil well that can be used to pollute. Be careful about the information you share online, be it period-tracking apps or ultrasound scans on social media. Look at who owns the major tech companies and their shareholders and ask yourself, do I want those guys knowing about my period or in control of what the world knows about my health? Tread carefully.

7. Horizon scan

When you become focused on one problem with women's health you can miss others. I don't want to sound too much like a feminist T-shirt here, but you have to outsmart the patriarchy, and doing this involves horizon scanning: what are the major challenges in the world and how will they impact on women's health? The most obvious, for example, would be climate change. Climate change is already having a direct impact on women's health in terms of food insecurity (for every ten malnourished men in the world there are eleven malnourished women), environmental disaster risk and management, and who is to blame for climate change. One of the biggest myths about climate change is it is being driven by population growth, notably the reproductive capabilities of the poor. The ability of women and children to survive pregnancy and childbirth are not to blame for climate change. But for some politicians and ecofascists, women's health is a great fall gal. Climate change is just one example, but there are multiple other issues – anti-microbial resistance (AMR), pandemic planning, non-communicable diseases in low-income countries – that are all relevant to women's health. As this book has shown, women's health has a powerful role to play in global politics, so how it is exploited will shift with the times.

8. Believe women

Change happens when women don't stay silent or hidden but talk to each other and believe each other. You overcome fear by knowing you are not alone but part of a wider movement across the world that has been fighting for change for women like you. We must forge political campaigns and movements to create change and break stigmas that divide us. When the world is not listening, women in Kenya, the US, UK and Argentina need other women to pay attention, to believe them and to amplify their voices to make people listen. Health workers and leaders share their stories with people like me to make sense of sick politics for readers like you. Women in poor countries need women in the US to lobby their politicians to stop gagging them. Women – *all* women – need to stick together and keep talking to each other. This is a solidarity politics that prioritises all of us over the individual.

The simplest thing you can do is believe women when they tell you they are sick, need money, have an idea, are being exploited or are in pain.

Worth the Effort

1. Do the obvious: how to send money and volunteer

Do the obvious. Send money. Volunteer. Because these two actions are seemingly obvious they are often dismissed as being piecemeal. There is a sexism to such dismissal, as if volunteering or giving money is women's work and therefore of less value, with less potential for significant change, or less radical. I would not say that to the volunteer driver who risks her own safety to drive women needing abortions across borders in the US, or the women I met in the community in Kenya who cared for people dying of AIDS. Voluntary work has forever been fundamental to women being able to access safe healthcare. As I explored earlier in the book, some work can be exploitative when it is unpaid, especially in systems with billions of aid money available to pay women. But not all voluntary work is exploitative. For example, every week since 2016 I have visited a woman who lives on her own and never leaves her house. I am a befriender volunteer for an age charity. I've had training, I take my role seriously and I give up my time (two hours, including walking to her house and back) as an unpaid volunteer. I am different to the carers who come into her house; they are paid for their labour and expertise (though it's worth noting that in the UK one in five of the people who report to modern slavery charity Unseen UK are carers like the ones who visit my friend). They should be paid carers: I am the unpaid volunteer who sits around chatting.

To identify the sort of voluntary work you want to do, think about the issues in this book that you are most affected by. If, for example, sexual and reproductive health is your thing, you could join an abortion support network as a clinic defender or phone line operator or, alternatively, if you want to get more women into leadership positions you could volunteer for organisations that engage in advocacy in a specific sector.

A question lots of friends ask me is where and how to spend money. I could write a lengthy appendix of organisations that want your cash, but these organisations, especially smaller ones, can change where they're operating, the work they're doing, the approach they take and may, by the time you're reading this, no longer align to your own specific interests or the sort of commitment you want to make. Big charities are easy to identify and send money to. Smaller organisations – which all my friends and family tend to ask me about – do require a bit more research. To do this, start by picking an issue, think about where the problem is the most acute and spend a good three hours researching different organisations. See if you can check their registration status, although this may not be suitable for all organisations. For example, a women's organisation may not register in Afghanistan since the Taliban restricted women's rights and organisations in 2022 – a lack of registration doesn't mean an organisation is dodgy, it may mean they're trying to stay safe. Crucially, check who else they may be partnered with and give/take money from. This last point is potentially the really big red flag. Some women's health organisations may present themselves as progressive on the first page of their website, but have regressive policies on safe abortion access, trans women, and/or comprehensive sex education. Checking out the language on these issues (see the 'Become a dog' section on dogwhistling above) and who they partner with offer a good indicator as to whether you want to give them money.

Once you have sent money, do not try to control how that money is spent or expect constant updates on how it has been spent. Trust that the person or organisation you are sending money to is putting it to good use. Always send money, not stuff. This especially applies in humanitarian contexts. For example, when people are displaced from their homes because of a crisis, there is a tendency for others to want to give clothes, blankets, baby formula and tents. While well-intended, this can in reality mean ill-fitting clothes, nowhere to store the formula and an abundance of tents when what people need is rent money for temporary accommodation and food. Money is always more useful and more flexible for organisations and individuals. It gives autonomy to the people you want to help.

Giving money and volunteering are of course short-term fillers for the ills in our politics and society. You should not have to give money to help someone set up an alternative rite of passage to FGM, or to send abortion pills over the phone, or organise a mother and baby kit. We should live in societies where these aspects of healthcare are seen as a public good, which we all contribute to through tax. But as long as some of these initiatives are illegal, woefully under-provided for or discriminated against they need money from other sources. I used not to give money, thinking in doing so I was letting the government ignore an issue, but then I realised the government didn't care about my political stance on this and people would keep voting for them, and my theory was all well and good for me but not helping the most vulnerable.

2. Build networks and be boring: changing your workplace

If you work in a health-based institution and want to advance change there are several things you can do. First, build a network of other women or like-minded people within the organisation. If you can't find anyone who is interested in gender equality, think about building networks outside your organisation. Attend conferences, talks, workshops and events where you can meet people who are experiencing the same issues and share tips on how to navigate them. This is not always possible when you are time and internet restricted, but the hybrid nature of these events makes them more accessible than before. Similarly, find your people on social media.

Second, know your labour laws and the norms and practices of the institution you work for. Knowing basic gender equality laws is useful for you in terms of your own rights, but also in advocating for the practices and priorities the organisation you work for should be following for everyone. One of the strongest tools you have regarding gender equality in institutions is knowing the rules and procedures and in what circumstances they apply. This will not necessarily make you popular. But it is effective. Depersonalise the topic and make it about institutional commitments. The more boring, the better.

Third, be an ally to all women. Seek out good mentors and be a good mentor in turn. Being a good mentor and ally means giving up your time; be realistic about how much time you can commit, and to how many people. Know when to reiterate the point a woman has made and attribute that good point to her. Never, ever, ever steal a woman's (or anyone's for that matter) idea or accomplishment and pass it off as your own. Look for opportunities to promote women you work with. Amplify women's voices inside and outside work. If a woman is being trolled on social media, offer to screenshot, block, report and delete all content so there is a record but she doesn't have to see it. With their consent, say something if someone is being bullied, harassed or abused in the workplace. If you are senior or in a position of power, stick your neck out for other women. Sometimes being an ally is shutting up and stepping back and knowing when to do so. Don't be hard on yourself if you don't always get it right, but do learn and apologise (properly, with no *ifs* or *buts*, e.g. 'Sorry if you thought I offended you'). A simple 'I am sorry for what I did and how it affected you'.

3. Employ a team of gender experts, and resource them properly

Gender experts are great at flagging issues that institutions with inequality problems are often blind to. However, for gender experts to do their job properly they need:

1. Proper resources, a clear budget line and a mandate to do their job.
2. A team. A single person will always be overworked.
3. Clear expectations as to what the role involves. Being a gender expert does not mean they have to appear in every picture, sit in every meeting or take the minutes. Your gender expert is not your organisation's EDI (equality, diversity and inclusion) lead. A gender expert and an EDI lead are not the same thing, so do not just tack gender expert onto the EDI lead's job and vice versa.
4. To be valued among colleagues as much as science, medicine and public health.
5. To be experts on gender inequality, with clear experience and expertise on gender and health.

If you have the opportunity to work as a gender expert within a health organisation (or any organisation, for that matter), ensure that the organisation meets the above five criteria before you sign the contract, and that you get this in writing. You may really want the job, have already negotiated your salary (*always* negotiate your salary; no one is going to withdraw an offer if you ask for more) and feel uncomfortable making extra demands and therefore tell yourself it won't be that bad. Reader, it will be that bad. Best to get the uncomfortable stuff out the way first to signal your intent, your employer's commitment and know you're being set up to succeed.

4. Stop the exploitation of women and girls: building a campaign

This is the big one. Given this book is all about how women's health is exploited for political gain, one of the biggest things we need to change is the exploitation of women and girls. Here I want to set out three concrete priorities and what you can do to help reach them.

Pay women for their labour
The global community needs to recognise and reward health and care labour, and value the skills the predominantly feminised health workforce has. This requires more than special days or token prizes: health workers need to be paid enough money to live and thrive in their jobs.

The first way of doing this is for current paid health workers to join a trade union. Unions are only as strong as their members; the more members, and the more active the members, the more influence and negotiation power they have with employers to get a better wage. If you are not a member of a union, you can still help them by monitoring laws that try to block the powers of unions, and show support for any industrial action by standing on a picket line (even in extreme weather, picket lines tend to be very friendly and fun spaces), give money to a solidarity fund and beep your horn when you drive past union members outside their place of work. Paint a picture, wear a sticker, like all the social media posts: it all adds up. Industrial action undertaken by health-worker unions is contentious because the stakes of withdrawing their labour can be high. However, during most periods of industrial action, health unions spend a lot of time planning and putting into place emergency provision to avoid harm. And remember, most union members want to do their jobs and not take action; they also lose money when they do. Given everything you've read about burnout, low pay and working conditions in the health sector, think about where any complaint should be targeted, with employers, health sector leaders and governments, not the workers themselves.

The second issue is the exploitation of unpaid health workers seen in Chapter 9 – community health workers, peer educators, data entry clerks – on whom the billion-dollar aid industry for health depends. The WHO and ILO recommends paying care workers. The US government acknowledges this is an issue. Primary health advocates emphasise the need for change. Sustainable Development Goal 5 'strongly recommends paying community health workers'. And yet, there is very little action or money. Payment of health workers needs to be a condition of *any* health project, regardless of size. Donors need to include health-worker payment as a core condition of funding. Governments need to cost such payments into any primary health and care strategy. We need to build a campaign to demand every aid donor and every government and private body commit to paying community health workers, to Pay Her Now. Some health groups are already pushing for change on these issues, but such work needs funding. This requires one of the biggest funders of health programmes – the US government, the Bill & Melinda Gates Foundation, the

UK, the EU – and a major government in the global south – India, South Africa, Brazil – to take a stand, factor in the costs and Pay Her Now. It needs citizens like you to demand they take a stand on this issue.

Stop fundraising campaigns that use images of children

Fundraising campaigns, specifically campaigns where the person in the image can be identified, should not include images of children. Stop giving money to any organisation that uses these images. When you see these images on your social media feed, write a comment asking for the image to be taken down. Petition key organisations to remove existing images from their websites and to make a commitment to no longer use such images. If you work for an organisation that uses these images, find like-minded people who are also concerned (they will exist!) and approach the head of the organisation as a unified group. The good news is, campaigners are already doing a lot of work on this, but numbers and more energy always helps. Running campaigns and calling out abuse is important work, but can be exhausting: new committed people and energy are crucial to building momentum and making this momentum sustainable so that the campaign doesn't end when those who started it become overwhelmed by the work.

If you lead a major medical humanitarian or global health organisation, undertake a review of your organisation's use of images. If you identify a problem, be transparent and set out a course of action to remedy the past and set a clear intent for the future. You have the profile and potential to develop best practice across the international community should you choose to.

If you are a designer selecting images for health policy reports, strategies, updates or websites for *any* organisation, start using pictures of people who actually represent your leadership and workforce instead of the more progressive image you like to present to the world. Nothing rankles more than seeing women of colour on the front of a policy report for an institution that underpays and undervalues women of colour. I know it would make policy documents boring and unappealing to people who read it, but putting the executive team on the cover of every official document would be a good transparency tool – yep, still all men! – and if such covers are unappealing, or unrepresentative of the people the institution wants to target, you can say the same for the leadership.

End sexual abuse and exploitation by health workers
The United Nations has a zero-tolerance approach to sexual abuse and exploitation, and has a clear standard of conduct. As you have read, zero tolerance means very little in practice, and mechanisms are often established after the fact. Ending sexual abuse and exploitation entirely across large organisations may be impossible, but reducing the extent of the problem is definitely possible.

The case of sexual exploitation, abuse and harassment in the DRC from Chapter 6 is a good example of this. People in the DRC working in the Ebola response were aware of what was happening, but nothing was done about it. Then women spoke out. Survivors were heard when a couple of journalists from Europe were told about their stories from their contacts in the DRC. Once these stories came out, the WHO had to listen. When change was slow in the WHO, a network of people, including investigative journalists, employees of global health institutions, activists and academics like me started talking to each other to share information and contacts and press for change. When activists became frustrated with a lack of progress in the WHO they started to talk to governments, and when governments did not listen they targeted key politicians they knew were sympathetic to women's issues. Keep talking, keep asking, keep working together.

Change first requires a reset in thinking on where the risk is: the danger is not (only) out there but in the institutions that are supposed to help, the supposed good guys. Second, any strategy, training or policy on sexual abuse, exploitation and harassment has to focus internally as well as externally. Every staff member of a major foreign organisation working in another country should undergo training on standards and codes of conduct and be aware of anonymous reporting structures. This training should not be a one-off, but held regularly and adapted to the relevant country contexts. An emergency is not an excuse to ignore this: emergencies create contexts with a high risk of abuse, exploitation and harassment and therefore such training is even more important. Third, every institution should have an up-to-date, independent, well-resourced strategy and reporting mechanism that is clearly communicated and tailored to the countries they work in. These communications should be in the appropriate languages and format. For example, posters in one language in the WHO country office in the DRC won't cut it: the communication has to be where the people and survivors are. Fourth, the pathway to how cases are investigated, timelines and outcomes should be transparent in training and in the code of conduct for all staff in the institution. Finally, the final report and decision on any case of sexual exploitation and abuse must be made by an independent agency or organisation. As the issues with the WHO in this book show, locating these powers with the director-general when the director-general is compromised is highly problematic. With any major case of sexual abuse and exploitation, the head of the organisation should take accountability and resign, as in the case of Oxfam and UNAIDS.

If you work within a health organisation, review the current sexual abuse, exploitation and harassment guidance within your agency. If you work for a UN agency, work with the UN special co-ordinator on improving prevention and response mechanisms. Use the evidence in this book and the reports from the DRC as a warning as to what can happen if your agency does not act or you are batted away with the usual excuses of 'no time/budget for that'. If you suspect a case, report it. If you've reported a case and there is no action, leak it to journalists.

To leak to journalists, see who has been reporting on similar issues and reach out to them. Sometimes this does not progress immediately, but it can be part of building a wider case against a person or agency so don't be disheartened. For example, several women spoke to reporters about an individual in a UN agency but the story didn't go anywhere. Years later, when high-profile cases related to the agency started to appear in the news, a network of women working in the field connected these survivors to journalists working on similar stories. This time the stories helped build a case against perpetrators and the agency in question. While it is disheartening to share a story that does not go anywhere at the time, part of the process of being believed is unfortunately about building networks of trust, critical mass and momentum. It is an unavoidable reality that, as with many high-profile cases, such as the Harvey Weinstein abuse, this can take years of frustrating inaction (during which perpetrators continue to abuse).

If you don't work for the UN and live in a country that contributes to the budget of health organisations such as the WHO, demand greater accountability for your tax money through your political representatives. This may not be the political representative for where you live, rather a politician that you know cares about these issues. Write to them, contact their office, meet them in their constituency hours. Politicians are really busy people, with competing demands on their time, so chances are they would not necessarily have heard of the issue you are telling them about. This does not mean they don't want to know about it. UN agencies depend on government money and the threat of financial withdrawal is the biggest lever donors have.

Aid-recipient countries also have leverage on these issues. Part of the mandate of key UN institutions such as the WHO is to work in countries with the greatest need: this is what they are paid to do. There are a range of health institutions and agencies wanting to give money to low- and middle-income countries. Aid-recipient countries have some potential to shop around for donors and organisations they want to work with. There is an unspoken divide in the foreign aid community between old-school donors from Europe and America and new types of donor from countries such as China. Old-school donors are worried that they will lose their influence if new donors take up the aid space: poorer countries can exploit this. If a particular donor does not account for actions on sexual exploitation and abuse, governments can ban them from a country until they have their house in order. This is a big card to play as it could have ripple effects for other international partners, e.g., if you chuck out one donor or organisation from your country, there is a risk that other countries may withhold aid until you relent. But first, I can't see donors doing this on clear cases of abuse and exploitation, and second, the threat in itself will have influence as long as the government in question briefs the press and other donors in the international community. This is a way in which aid-recipient countries can shame organisations into action.

5. Rethink foreign aid: how not to stay silent

I have argued in this book that women's health is at the centre of international diplomacy, foreign aid, conflict and global institution building. It is not a neutral scientific space free from politics. It is highly politicised area, from which issues receive money, who is silenced, which dead bodies are counted and who is subject to violence, to who gets to lead and who does the front-line work. This is politics, not science. You can have all the scientific advancements in the world on women's health, but this will not help women unless you have a system of global politics that values women's health for what it is, rather than as a means to power.

A system that depends on the exploitation of women and girls and contradicts its own norms and values is not a good system. Neither is a system that is distorted by foreign gag rules, world leaders turning a blind eye to harm and health institutions that will do anything but take a woman leader or gender equality seriously. It is a system that does not work for women or their health needs. A myth used to silence women and overlook exploitation is the idea that if you call something out you risk damaging the whole sector by stopping the aid money flowing. This is bullshit and a silencing tactic. The billion-dollar aid industry for health cannot be undone by one woman or a movement of women speaking out, and if it is, then good: nothing needs more reform than the exploitative aid for health industry.

Keep calling it out. If someone blames you for destroying a billion-dollar industry – wow, what power you have! – ask them why they are defending an exploitative, rotten industry.

With every programme or initiative on women's health, ask the basic questions: who is being served? Whose interests do these initiatives represent? What is being prioritised? Who benefits and who loses out? And who is being sidelined or ignored?

We need to make political interests in women's health transparent. Transparency means holding governments and international organisations to account. We need to ask our representatives where our tax money goes and call them out when they buddy up with other politicians who think it is okay to sterilise women, not to pay them, to harass or exploit them. Transparency not only holds powerful actors to account, it also helps break stigma and shame. When we are transparent about how women experience ill health and the exploitation of women in addressing the world's health needs, we break the isolation of women thinking it is just happening to them.

Finally, progress in one area of women's health is often used to justify exploitation or inaction on another. This starts with classic deflection tactics, where you ask a question about health-worker pay and receive an answer about how much money the government or donor has invested in the health system. Or you ask about why women were ignored in COVID-19 planning and you are informed about someone's years working on maternal health. When deflection stops working there is the shift to the 'are you not satisfied?' questions: are you not satisfied that we now pay health workers/ have 30 per cent of women on our board/sacked the rapist/ have a menopause strategy? – simple answer being, thanks but nope. This shift plays on two ideas: first, that women and girls should be grateful for a seat at the table, to be paid the same as men or not be harassed or exploited at work, and that to speak out means you are not sufficiently grateful; and second, that people who deliver change deserve praise, or what feminists with characteristic humour call biscuit-seeking behaviour ('well done for promoting the over-qualified woman, have a biscuit'). You don't have to be grateful to people and institutions for doing the right thing and adhering to the global standards that they often set.

Mid-way through writing this book, I received a message from one of the students I taught some years back. She hadn't known anything about global health politics until she took my class in the third year of her undergraduate degree. She was messaging me as she wanted me to know that my module, and everything she had learned about maternal mortality and gender inequality in health, had inspired her to make a difference, and she had decided to train as a midwife. She thought about what she could do and how it would fit with her interests and passions and she did it. It is one of the best messages I've ever received. As the amazing women in this book show, you are not alone in being sick of the way women's health is used for political gain, and regardless of the huge power structures we are up against, if you want to, there is always something you can do to stop women from dying when they don't have to.

Note on Sources

Research for this book involved 111 original interviews, which took place between 2019 and 2022 in the UK, US, Sierra Leone, Kenya and Palestine, and on Zoom/Teams/WhatsApp from my home in 2020. Some of the stories are drawn from my wider research on global health and previous 250-plus interviews conducted with health policy specialists, practitioners, health professionals, local authorities, patient groups, NGOs, community groups, militaries, UN agencies, women's groups and gender equality specialists around the world since 2005. In addition to these interviews I have reviewed every women and gender equality strategy of global health organisations pre- and post COVID-19, policy guidance, strategy documents and frameworks for specific health issues and topics, official aid funding, biographies, health budget allocations, political speeches and academic publications. Parts of the book are drawn from my observations as a participant in key meetings and events, particularly around Ebola, HIV/AIDS and COVID-19. I was one of the founding members of the global Gender and COVID-19 Working Group, and produced real-time research with colleagues during the pandemic; where relevant I draw from these experiences. Where I detail a meeting that I was not in, I have consulted meeting minutes (where available), watched videos of the meeting, read secondary sources or, where possible, discussed it with people who were there.

The names of people in the book have been changed, and the only exception to this is if the person is in the public eye, e.g. a politician, prominent civil servant, head of a UN agency; is named in a public document; has told their stories on the public record; or has specifically requested to have their name published. The easy way to tell if a name has been changed is if I just use a first name. Everyone I spoke to was aware of why I was talking to them and consented to be included in the book.

I deliberately chose not to interview heads of state, UN agencies or leading politicians for the book. In my experience, these interviews require a lot of resources to organise and produce little new insight while the person is still in office. Such leaders also have a lot of representation in other spaces (and in some cases their own books), and I wanted to showcase and focus on the women we don't hear from as much, but for me are more important and fundamental to health in the world. Instead, I looked at the public statements, speeches, social media, books and press releases of more senior leaders to ensure they are still represented in the book in their own words.

I have prioritised narrative over academic citations and debates within the book. Where possible I have flagged key books, authors and research projects in the main text. A full list of sources for each chapter can be found in 'Sources' at the end of the book.

Note of Thanks

Huge thank you to everyone who took the time to talk to me for this book, trusted me with information or took the time to explain things at different points in my career. Lots of the people who appear in this book are very busy, trying their best in complex political systems or keeping members of their family and community alive and I am incredibly grateful for any time they have offered me, the follow-up emails with links to further information and new introductions. The aim of all my work is to be able to explain how politics shapes inequality and injustice in the world in order for us to do something about it, and for people to feel less alone or forgotten – all of which depends on people trusting me and sharing stories and what they know.

This book was made possible by research funding from the Leverhulme Trust's Philip Leverhulme Prize. The Philip Leverhulme Prize is an absolute gift and I am enormously grateful to the Leverhulme Trust for being so understanding and supportive as my initial project twisted and turned in response to COVID-19.

Sara E. Davies, Laleh Khalili and Joanne Yao read the first draft of the book. I am so grateful for their time, and that the initial draft got through the first pass of such incredible women. Sara and Laleh have heard about this book for too long, and have been hugely encouraging throughout the process. Thank you Sharri Plonski for helping explain the different borders and walls of Palestine, Róisín Read for the advice on attacks on health workers, and the camaraderie, solidarity and inspiration from my QM buddies. Thanks to the organisers and audiences of the LSE annual Fred Halliday lecture and the University of Bristol's Gender Research Centre Annual Lecture for inviting me to present and test the ideas in this book. Melissa Slep provided excellent research assistance; her spreadsheets are a thing of wonder, as is her own work on sexual and reproductive justice. Thanks to Caterina Mazzilli and Kathrin Fischer for their great transcription work of my badly recorded interviews. Thank you to the wider community of women, gender and global health scholars and activists, especially the original Gender and COVID-19 working group, whom I think I spoke to more than my own family in 2020–21. Big love and gratitude for the fantastic students I've taught and learned so much from over the last decade; you continue to inspire and challenge me and my work.

Sick of It started as a convoluted academic book written during the blur of 2020–21 lockdowns. Duncan Bell suggested scrapping the academic version and writing a more accessible book, and he was right. Apologies to the scrapped manuscript sitting in an unloved folder. Massive thanks to Andrew Gordon at David Higham Associates for taking me and the book on, believing I could do this, and finding such a brilliant publisher. Thanks to Rose Tomaszewska who first got it, and Sarah Savitt who shaped it. Sarah is an absolute joy to work with – such a brilliant and generous editor and publisher. She pushed me and the book to be better than I could have imagined when I started. To build on the legacy of Virago is a privilege.

Final thanks to my family and friends – Becky, Gem, Cathy, Laura, Simukai, Jemima, Jamie, James, Lucy, Cat and Spark – who heard me go on (and on) about the book in endless loops of the parks of east London, and everyone at Move for doing so much for this woman's health. Big thanks to my mum, who took us in for four months during a particularly tricky time in the formation of the book and my home. My work can be pretty bleak and joyless at times, but my life is not. Kieran my partner and Bruce the dog are the best companions any writer could want, and their support, especially during the wild-eyed phase of the end of the project, has been incredible. I have to say this as this is the only part of the book one of them will read, but their ongoing support and love is the antidote.

This book is dedicated to the memory of my friend Peris Bosibori Onsongo, whom I met when I started asking questions about women's health in 2005, and who died far too young in 2023.

Sources

1: Soft Power and Healthwashing

1 Katia Savchuk (2014). 'How Rwanda went from genocide to global health model', *The World*, https://theworld.org/dispatches/globalpost-blogs/global-pulse/rwanda-genocide-global-health; Agnes Binagwaho et al. (2014). 'Rwanda 20 years on: investing in life', *Lancet* 384(9940): 371–5, https://www.thelancet.com/journals/lancet/article/PIIS0140-6736(14)60574-2/fulltext#seccestitle10.
2 Binagwaho et al. (2014). 'Rwanda 20 years on'.
3 Binagwaho et al. (2014). 'Rwanda 20 years on'.
4 Katia Savchuk (2014). 'Q&A with Paul Farmer: Rwanda as a healthcare success story', *The World*, https://theworld.org/dispatches/globalpost-blogs/global-pulse/paul-farmer-rwanda-healthcare-paul-farmer.
5 Binagwaho et al. (2014). 'Rwanda 20 years on'.
6 Katrina Manson (2015). 'Kagame seeks lasting economic miracle for Rwanda', *Financial Times*, https://www.ft.com/content/3cdd59b0-ded5-11e4-b9ec-00144feab7de.
7 Savchuk (2014). 'How Rwanda went from genocide to global health model'.
8 Savchuk (2014). 'Q&A with Paul Farmer: Rwanda as a healthcare success story'.
9 UN Women (2018). 'Revisiting Rwanda five years after record-breaking parliamentary elections', https://www.unwomen.org/en/news/stories/2018/8/feature-rwanda-women-in-parliament.
10 BBC News Africa (2015). 'How has Rwanda saved the lives of 590,000 children?', https://www.bbc.co.uk/news/world-africa-32438104; Richard Horton (2013). 'Offline: The Rwandan Miracle', *Lancet* 383(9889): 294, https://www.thelancet.com/journals/lancet/article/PIIS0140-6736(13)61608-6/fulltext.

11 Richard Horton (2013). 'Offline: The Rwandan Miracle', *Lancet* 383(9889): 294, https://www.thelancet.com/journals/lancet/article/PIIS0140-6736(13)61608-6/fulltext.

12 Horton (2013). 'Offline: The Rwandan Miracle'.

13 Binagwaho et al. (2014). 'Rwanda 20 years on'; Heidi Worley (2015). 'Rwanda's Success in Improving Mental Health', *PRB*, https://www.prb.org/resources/rwandas-success-in-improving-maternal-health/#:~:text=Rwanda's%20maternal%20mortality%20ratio%20decreased,deaths%20per%201%2C000%20live%20births.

14 Chunling Lu, Benjamin Cook and Chris Desmond (2017). 'Does foreign aid crowd out government investments? Evidence from rural health centres in Rwanda', *BMJ Global Health* 2:e000364, https://gh.bmj.com/content/2/3/e000364.

15 Enoch Randy Aikins and Alize le Roux (2023). 'Could FDI be Rwanda's lifeline as donors pull the plug?' Institute for Security Studies, https://issafrica.org/iss-today/could-fdi-be-rwandas-lifeline-as-donors-pull-the-plug#:~:text=Rwanda%20has%20received%20significant%20support,and%20Kenya%20with%20US%2460.

16 University of Global Health Equity (2023). 'Closing the Gender Gap in Global Health Science', https://ughe.org/closing-the-gender-gap-in-global-health-science.

17 Women Deliver (2023). https://womendeliver.org/.

18 Amnesty International (2023). 'Repression in post-genocide Rwanda', https://www.amnesty.org/en/latest/campaigns/2017/09/rwandas-repressive-tactics-silence-dissent-before-elections.

19 Michela Wrong (2021). *Do Not Disturb: The Story of a Political Murder and an African Regime Gone Bad*, London: Harper Collins.

20 Michela Wrong (2021). *Do Not Disturb: The Story of a Political Murder and an African Regime Gone Bad*, London: Harper Collins; David Himbara (2019). 'Kagame Finally Admits He Had Sendashonga Assassinated' *Medium*, https://medium.com/@david.himbara_27884/kagame-finally-admits-he-had-sendashonga-assassinated-aeb120478879.

21 Wrong, *Do Not Disturb*.

22 Richard Horton (2016). 'Offline: the King and his courtiers', *Lancet* 387 (1800), https://www.thelancet.com/pdfs/journals/lancet/PIIS0140-6736(16)30309-9.pdf.

23 Laurie Garrett (2018). 'Rwanda: not the official narrative', *Lancet* 392 (10151), 909-912, https://www.thelancet.com/pdfs/journals/lancet/PIIS0140-6736(18)32124-X.pdf.

24 Agnes Binagwaho, Ruton Hinda and Edward Mills (2019). 'Rwanda and revisionist history', *Lancet* 393(10169): 319–20, https://www.thelancet.com/journals/lancet/article/PIIS0140-6736(19)30121-7/fulltext.

25 Jessica Moody (2022). 'How Rwanda Became Africa's Policeman', *Foreign Policy*, https://foreignpolicy.com/2022/11/21/ how-rwanda-became-africas-policeman.

2: The Aid Boom and Saving Mothers

1 Global Burden of Disease 2020 Health Financing Collaborator Network (2021). 'Tracking development assistance for health and for COVID-19: a review of development assistance, out-of-pocket, and other private spending on health for 204 countries and territories, 1990–2050', *Lancet* 398(1): 317–43, https://www.thelancet.com/action/ showPdf?pii=S0140-6736%2821%2901258-7.

2 Commonwealth Secretariat (1989), *Engendering Adjustment for the 1990s: Report of a Commonwealth Expert Group on Women and Structural Adjustment*, London, 31.

3 Vandita Mishra (2022). 'If you invest in women, they invest in everyone else: Melinda French Gates Exclusive', *Indian Express*, https://www.youtube.com/watch?v=3vlQ1yjMdoA.

4 Joseph Hanlon, Armando Barrientos and David Hulme (2010). *Just Give Money to the Poor: The Development Revolution From the Global South*, Sterling, VA: Kumarian Press.

5 Joseph Hanlon, Armando Barrientos and David Hulme (2010). *Just Give Money to the Poor: The Development Revolution From the Global South*, Sterling, VA: Kumarian Press.

6 OECD. 'Sector 1.3 Population Policies/Programmes and Reproductive Health', https://stats.oecd.org/qwids/#?x=3&y=6&f= 2:262,4:1,7:2,9:85,5:4,8:85,1:1&q=2:262+4:1+7:2+9:85+5:4+8:85+ 1:1+3:21,22,23,24,26,27,28,29,30,31,32,33,35,36,37,38,39+6:200 5,2006,2007,2008,2009,2010,2011,2012,2013,2014,2015,2016,2 017,2018,2019 (accessed July 2023).

7 UNAIDS (2003). *2003 AIDS Epidemic Update*, https://data. unaids.org/pub/report/2003/2003_epiupdate_en.pdf.

8 OECD. 'Sector 1.2 Noncommunicable diseases', https://stats.oecd. org/qwids/#?x=3&y=6&f=2:262,4:1,7:2,9:85,5:4,8:85,1:1&q= 2:262+4:1+7:2+9:85+5:4+8:85+1:1+3:21,22,23,24,26,27,28,29,3 0,31,32,33,35,36,37,38,39+6:2005,2006,2007,2008,2009,2010, 2011,2012,2013,2014,2015,2016,2017,2018,2019 (accessed July 2023).

9 UNICEF (2021). 'Maternal Mortality', https://data.unicef.org/ topic/maternal-health/maternal-mortality/#:~:text=Levels%20 of%20maternal%20mortality,2000%20to%20295%2C000%20 in%202017.

10 UNAIDS (2016). 'Children and HIV: Factsheet', https://www.

unaids.org/sites/default/files/media_asset/FactSheet_Children_
en.pdf.

3: Hard Power and the Global Gag Rule

1 MSI Choices. 'The impact of the global gag rule on frontline
reproductive healthcare', https://www.msichoices.org/media/3884/
msi-briefing-impact-of-the-ggr-on-reproductive-healthcare.pdf.
2 Alex Gray (2017). 'These countries are pledging to fill the funding
gap left by America's controversial "global gag rule"', *World
Economic Forum*, https://www.weforum.org/agenda/2017/03/
global-gag-rule-abortion-family-planning.
3 Z. Kmietowicz (2019). 'Abortion: US "global gag rule" is killing
women and girls, says report', *BMJ 365*: l4118, https://www.bmj.
com/content/365/bmj.l4118.
4 Zara Ahmed (2020). 'The Unprecedented Expansion of the Global
Gag Rule: Trampling Rights, Health and Free Speech', Guttmacher
Institute, https://www.guttmacher.org/gpr/2020/04/unprecedented-
expansion-global-gag-rule-trampling-rights-health-and-free-speech.
5 Nina Brooks, Eran Bendavid and Grant Miller (2019). 'USA aid
policy and induced abortion in sub-Saharan Africa: an analysis
of the Mexico City Policy', *Lancet Global Health* 7(8): E1046-
E1053, https://www.thelancet.com/journals/langlo/article/
PIIS2214-109X(19)30267-0/fulltext.
6 UNFPA Zimbabwe (2022). 'What we do: Sexual and
Reproductive Health', https://zimbabwe.unfpa.org/en/topics/
sexual-reproductive-health-5.
7 International Campaign for Women's Right to Safe Abortion
(2019). 'Malawi – Abortion law reform bill in Malawi supported by
religious leaders – again', https://www.safeabortionwomensright.
org/news/malawi-abortion-law-reform-bill-in-malawi-supported-
by-religious-leaders-again.
8 Center for Reproductive Rights (2023). 'The World's Abortion
Laws', https://reproductiverights.org/maps/worlds-abortion-laws.
9 Center for Reproductive Rights (2023). 'The World's Abortion
Laws'.
10 Guttmacher Institute (2017). 'Abortion and Postabortion care in
Malawi', https://www.guttmacher.org/fact-sheet/abortion-malawi.
11 International Campaign for Women's Right to Safe Abortion
(2019). 'Malawi – Abortion law reform bill'.
12 Lameck Masina (2021). 'Malawi Parliament Withdraws Abortion
Rights Bill after Objections', *Voice of America*, https://www.
voanews.com/a/africa_malawi-parliament-withdraws-abortion-
rights-bill-after-objections/6207221.html.

13 AMECEA Social Communications (2017). 'Malawi: Let's call for a referendum on abortion bill – Archbishop Msusa appeals', Association of Member Episcopal Conference in Eastern Africa, https://communications.amecea.org/index.php/2017/12/02/malawi-lets-call-for-a-referendum-on-abortion-bill-archbishop-msusa-appeals.

14 Crux (2017). 'Catholic archbishop challenges Malawi's leaders on abortion law', https://cruxnow.com/global-church/2017/12/catholic-archbishop-challenges-malawis-leaders-abortion-law.

15 An excellent academic article on this is Elżbieta Korolczuk and Agnieszka Graff (2018). 'Gender as "Ebola from Brussels": the anticolonial frame and the rise of illiberal populism', *Signs*, 43(4): 797–821. https://www.journals.uchicago.edu/doi/abs/10.1086/696691?journalCode=signs.

16 CHANGE (2020). 'A Powerful Force: US Global Health Assistance and Sexual and Reproductive Health and Rights in Malawi', https://fosfeminista.org/wp-content/uploads/2022/04/Change_Malawi_Web_Pages.pdf.

17 CHANGE (2020). 'A Powerful Force'.

18 US Congress, S.368 – Global Health, Empowerment and Rights Act, 116th Congress (2019–2020), https://www.congress.gov/bill/116th-congress/senate-bill/368/text?r=477&s=3.

19 The White House (2021). 'Memorandum on Protecting Women's Health at Home and Abroad', https://www.whitehouse.gov/briefing-room/presidential-actions/2021/01/28/memorandum-on-protecting-womens-health-at-home-and-abroad.

4: Checkpoints, Blockades, Bombs and Pregnant Women

1 Juzoor Foundation for Health and Social Development (2005). 'Giving Birth @ The Check Point'.

2 UNHCR (2008). 'Palestinian pregnant women giving birth at Israeli checkpoints – HRC seventh session', https://www.un.org/unispal/document/auto-insert-186867.

3 UNHCR (2008). 'Palestinian pregnant women giving birth at Israeli checkpoints'.

4 Hammoudeh, Doaa, Coast, Ernestina, Lewis, David, Rabaia, Yoke, Leone, Tiziana and Giacaman, Rita (2017) 'Age of despair or age of hope? Palestinian women's perspectives on midlife health'. *Social Science & Medicine* . ISSN 0277-9536

5 Damien Gayle (2023). 'How bombings, blockades and import bans caused Gaza's water system to crumble', *Guardian*, https://www.theguardian.com/world/2023/oct/25/how-bombings-blockades-and-import-bans-caused-gaza-water-system-to-crumble.

6   WHO (2022). '15 years of Gaza blockade and barriers to health access', http://www.emro.who.int/images/stories/palestine/ documents/15-Years-Gaza-Blockade-Factsheet.pdf?ua=1&ua=1; WHO (2022). '15 years of blockade and health in Gaza'; http:// www.emro.who.int/images/stories/palestine/documents/15_years_ of_blockade_and_health_in-gaza.pdf?ua=1.

7   Tiziana Leone et al. (2019). 'Maternal and child access to care and intensity of conflict in the occupied Palestinian territory: a pseudo-longitudinal analysis (2000–2014)', *Conflict and Health* 13(36), https://conflictandhealth.biomedcentral.com/articles/10.1186/ s13031-019-0220-2.

8   WHO (2020). 'Health conditions in the occupied Palestinian territory, including east Jerusalem, and in the occupied Syrian Golan', Agenda Item 17, Seventy-Third World Health Assembly A73/15, https://apps.who.int/gb/ebwha/pdf_files/WHA73/ A73_15-en.pdf.

9   UNFPA (2020). *National Maternal Mortality Report 2020*, https:// palestine.unfpa.org/sites/default/files/pub-pdf/national_maternal_ mortality_report_2020_0.pdf.

10 Marie E. Thoma and Eugene R. Declercq (2022). 'Research letter: All-cause Maternal Mortality in the US Before vs During the COVID-19 Pandemic', *JAMA Network Open* 5(6) e2219133, https://jamanetwork.com/journals/jamanetworkopen/ fullarticle/2793640.

11 OCHA (2019). 'Mothers at risk: limited access to medicine and family planning services compromises maternal health in Gaza', https://www.ochaopt.org/content/mothers-risk-limited-access-medicine-and-family-planning-services-compromises-maternal.

12 UNFPA (2020). *National Maternal Mortality Report 2020*.

13 Larissa Fast and Roisin Read (2022). 'Using Data to Create Change? Interrogating the role of Data in Ending Attacks on Healthcare', *International Studies Review* 24(3), https://academic.oup.com/isr/article/24/3/ viac026/6593873?searchresult=1&login=false.

14 WHO (2022). 'Surveillance System for Attacks on Health Care: Ukraine', https://extranet.who.int/ssa/Index.aspx.

15 Ludvig Foghammar et al. (2016). 'Challenges in researching violence affecting health service delivery in complex security environments', *Social Science and Medicine* 162: 219–26, https:// www.sciencedirect.com/science/article/pii/S0277953616301393.

16 Swedish Red Cross/Jessica Cadesky (2015). *Study on Access to Health Care During Armed Conflict and Other Emergencies: Examining Violence Against Health Care from a Gender Perspective*, https://healthcareindanger.org/wp-content/ uploads/2015/12/report_-_study_on_hcidg_src_tryck.pdf.

5: Selling Trauma

1 Susan Sontag (2003). *Regarding the Pain of Others*, London: Penguin Random House.
2 Akanksha Mehta (2019). 'Teaching Gender, Race, Sexuality: Reflections on Feminist Pedagogy', *Kohl Journal* 5(1), https:// kohljournal.press/reflections-feminist-pedagogy; bell hooks (1992); 'Eating the other: desire and resistance', in *Black Looks: Race and Representation*, Boston, MA: South End Press.
3 WHO (2023). 'Cervical Cancer', https://www.who.int/news-room/ fact-sheets/detail/cervical-cancer.
4 Benjamin Chesterton (2021). 'Olivia Arthur – now can we talk about Magnum Photos and child abuse?', https://www.duckrabbit. info/blog/2021/01/olivia-arthur-now-can-we-talk-about-magnum- photos-and-child-abuse.
5 MSF (2023). 'Who we are', https://msf.org.uk/who-we-are.
6 MSF Child Protection Inquiry (2022). 'Letter to the Board of Médecins Sans Frontières/Doctors Without Borders', https:// msfchildprotect.wordpress.com/2022/05/24/letter.
7 David Batty (2022). 'Médecins San Frontières condemned for "profiting from exploitative images"', *Guardian*, https://www. theguardian.com/global-development/2022/may/25/medecins- sans-frontieres-condemned-for-profiting-from-exploitative-images; David Batty (2022). 'Médecins Sans Frontières pulls images of teenage rape survivor after outcry', *Guardian*, https://www. theguardian.com/world/2022/may/23/medecins-sans-frontieres- pulls-images-of-teenage-survivor-after-outcry.
8 MSF (2022). 'MSF Heads of Communications Commit to Tackle Problematic Imagery', https://msf.org.au/article/ statements-opinion/msf-heads-communications-commit-tackle- problematic-imagery; MSF (2022). 'MSF International President responds to photo ethics concerns', https://www.msf.org/ msf-international-president-responds-photo-ethics-concerns.

6: Sexual Exploitation, Abuse, Harassment and the UN

1 WHO (2018). 'Ebola – Hope is at the end of the tunnel in Mangina (East of the DRC)', https://www.afro.who.int/news/ ebola-hope-end-tunnel-mangina-east-drc.
2 WHO (2020). 'Ebola Virus Disease: Democratic Republic of Congo. External Situation Report 88', https://www.who.int/ publications/i/item/ebola-virus-disease-democratic-republic-of- congo-external-situation-report-88-2019.

3   WHO (2021). Final Report of the Independent Commission (28 September 2021), https://cdn.who.int/media/docs/default- source/ethics/ic- final- report- 28092021- en- version. pdf?sfvrsn=fef409a0_9&download=true.

4   WHO (2021). Final Report of the Independent Commission.

5   WHO (2021). Final Report of the Independent Commission.

6   Maria Cheng and Al-Hadji Kudra Maliro (2021). 'Panel finds 80 alleged abuse cases tied to WHO's Congo work', *Associated Press,* https://apnews.com/article/business-health-united-nations-world-health-organization-ebola-virus-36ceb41d266190d149a74e400332e1ed.

7   Jasmine-Kim Westendorf and Louise Searle (2017). 'Sexual exploitation and abuse in peace operations: trends, policy responses and future directions', *International Affairs* 93(2): 365–87, https://academic.oup.com/ia/article/93/2/365/2982811?login=true.

8   Megan Daigle, Sarah Martin and Henri Myrttinen (2021). '"Stranger Danger" and the Gendered/Racialized Construction of Threats in Humanitarianism', *Journal of Humanitarian Affairs* 2(3), https://www.manchesteropenhive.com/view/journals/jha/2/3/article-p4.xml?body=pdf.

9   Charity Commission for England and Wales (2019). *Inquiry Report: Summary Findings and Conclusions: Oxfam,* https://assets.publishing.service.gov.uk/government/uploads/system/uploads/attachment_data/file/807943/Inquiry_Report_summary_findings_and_conclusions_Oxfam.pdf.

10 Cathy Newman (2018). 'Oxfam whistleblower: allegations of rape and sex in exchange for aid', *Channel 4 News*, https://www.channel4.com/news/oxfam-whistleblower-allegations-of-rape-and-sex-in-exchange-for-aid.

11 Charity Commission for England and Wales (2019). *Inquiry Report: Summary Findings and Conclusions: Oxfam.*

12 Charity Commission for England and Wales (2019). *Inquiry Report: Summary Findings and Conclusions: Oxfam.*

13 Sean O'Neill (2018). 'Oxfam in Haiti: "It was like a Caligula orgy with prostitutes in Oxfam T-shirts"', *The Times*, https://www.thetimes.co.uk/article/oxfam-in-haiti-it-was-like-a-caligula-orgy-with-prostitutes-in-oxfam-T-shirts-p32wlk0rp.

14 Kevin Rawlinson (2018). 'Oxfam chief steps down after charity's sexual abuse scandal', *Guardian*, https://www.theguardian.com/world/2018/may/16/oxfam-head-mark-goldring-steps-down-sexual-abuse-scandal; Decca Aitkenhead (2018). 'Oxfam boss Mark Goldring: "Anything we say is being manipulated. We've been savaged"', *Guardian*, https://www.theguardian.com/world/2018/feb/16/oxfam-boss-mark-goldring-anything-we-say-is-being-manipulated-weve-been-savaged.

15 Nicola Slawson (2018). 'Oxfam government funding cut off after Haiti scandal', *Guardian*, https://www.theguardian.com/world/2018/feb/16/oxfam-government-funding-cut-off-after-haiti-scandal.

16 Maria Cheng and Al-Hadji Kudra Maliro (2021). 'Internal emails reveal WHO knew of sex abuse claims in the Congo', Associated Press, https://apnews.com/article/united-nations-europe-ebola-virus-entertainment-coronavirus-pandemic-d14715ba3653753d7c1f122f8aea79de.

17 Cheng and Maliro (2021). 'Internal emails reveal WHO knew of sex abuse claims'.

18 Cheng and Maliro (2021). 'Internal emails reveal WHO knew of sex abuse claims'.

19 Maria Cheng and Al-Hadji Kudra Maliro (2023). '"An absurdity": Experts slam WHO excusal of sex misconduct', Associated Press, https://apnews.com/article/crime-democratic-republic-of-the-congo-united-nations-niger-world-health-organization-b90517846748b161983350ec0c5296ca.

20 Simon Manley (2023). Tweet @SimonManleyFCDO, https://twitter.com/SimonManleyFCDO/status/1620504489039101952/photo/2.

21 Women in Global Health (2022). 'Her Story: Ending Sexual Violence and Harassment of Women Health Workers', https://womeningh.org/healthtoo.

22 Sarah Newey (2023). 'Top WHO scientist suspended amid claims of misogynistic p---ing circle', *Telegraph*, https://www.telegraph.co.uk/global-health/women-and-girls/top-who-scientist-suspended-amid-claims-misogynistic-pssing; Maria Cheng (2023). 'WHO knew of past sexual misconduct claim against doctor', Associated Press, https://apnews.com/article/politics-health-sexual-misconduct-berlin-fiji-fbbfa601f5dd9987ba2c011ce2d91d01; Al-Hadji Kudra Maliro and Maria Cheng (2023). '"Shame for WHO": victim of sex misconduct slams UN response', Associated Press, https://apnews.com/article/politics-sexual-misconduct-united-nations-world-health-organization-9bd4345598eae58cf8ce660653bd5dba.

23 Mick Krever (2018). 'UN agency chief to step down after damning report on culture of sexual harassment', *CNN*, https://edition.cnn.com/2018/12/14/world/michel-sidibe-unaids-into/index.html.

24 Udani Samarasekera (2022). *WHO sexual abuse allegations: 6 months on*, The Lancet, Volume 399, Issue 10333, 1372.

7: Attacking Health Workers, Normalising Violence Against Women

1 Royal College of Nursing (2021). 'RCN position on work related violence in health and social care', https://www.rcn.

org.uk/About-us/Our-Influencing-work/Position-statements/
rcn-position-on-work-related-violence-in-health-and-social-care.
2 Royal College of Nursing (2021). 'RCN position on work related
   violence in health and social care'.
3 Royal College of Nursing (2021). 'RCN position on work related
   violence in health and social care'.
4 WHO (2023). 'Preventing violence against health workers', https://
   www.who.int/activities/preventing-violence-against-health-workers.
5 International Labour Organization, International Council
   of Nurses, World Health Organization and Public Services
   International (2002). *Framework guidelines for addressing
   workplace violence in the health sector/Joint Programme on
   Workplace Violence in the Health Sector*, https://apps.who.int/iris/
   handle/10665/42617.
6 Brandi Leach and Michael Whitmore (2019). 'Is Training for
   NHS Staff to Manage Workplace Violence Effective?,' RAND
   Corporation, https://www.rand.org/blog/2019/09/is-training-for-
   nhs-staff-to-manage-workplace-violence.html.
7 Lisa A. Wolf, Altair M. Delao and Cydne Perhats (2014). 'Nothing
   Changes, Nobody Cares: Understanding the Experience of
   Emergency Nurses Physically or Verbally Assaulted While Providing
   Care', *Journal of Emergency Nursing*, 40(4): 305–10, https://www.
   jenonline.org/article/S0099-1767%2813%2900561-8/fulltext.
8 Wolf, Delao, Perhats (2014). 'Nothing changes, Nobody cares'.
9 International Labour Organization et al. (2002). *Framework
   guidelines for addressing workplace violence in the health sector/
   Joint Programme on Workplace Violence in the Health Sector*,
   https://www.ilo.org/global/topics/safety-and-health-at-work/
   resources-library/training/WCMS_108542/lang--en/index.htm.
10 International Labour Organization et al. (2002). *Framework
   guidelines*.
11 Asha S. George et al. (2020). 'Violence against female health
   workers is tip of iceberg of gender power imbalances', *BMJ* 371:
   m3546, https://www.bmj.com/content/371/bmj.m3546.
12 No Silence on ED Violence (2022), https://stopedviolence.org/
   resources.
13 Sai Balasubramanian (2021). 'Violence Against Healthcare Workers
   Is A Growing Problem', *Forbes*, https://www.forbes.com/sites/
   saibala/2021/04/29/violence-against-healthcare-workers-is-a-growing-
   problem/?sh=3dc68f32446c; No Silence on ED Violence (2023).
14 No Silence on ED Violence (2023); Wolf, Delao, Perhats (2014).
   'Nothing changes, Nobody cares'.
15 BBC News (2020). 'Salford Royal Infirmary patient jailed for
   NHS worker juice row attack', https://www.bbc.com/news/
   uk-england-manchester-52441325.

16 David Batty (2023). 'Approach to tackling violence raises concern among NHS England staff', *Guardian*, https://www.theguardian.com/society/2023/may/23/approach-to-tackling-violence-raises-concern-among-nhs-england-staff.

17 Batty (2023). 'Approach to tackling violence raises concern among NHS England staff'.

18 ICRC (2020). 'ICRC: 600 violent incidents recorded against health care providers, patients due to COVID-19', https://www.icrc.org/en/document/icrc-600-violent-incidents-recorded-against-healthcare-providers-patients-due-COVID-19.

19 Rebecca L. Root (2021). 'Health workers in India, Mexico saw most COVID-19-related violence in 2020', Devex, https://www.devex.com/news/health-workers-in-india-mexico-saw-most-COVID-19-related-violence-in-2020-99211.

20 Aatmika Nair et al. (2021). 'Solving systemic violence against healthcare workers in India', *BMJ Opinion*, https://blogs.bmj.com/bmj/2021/10/04/solving-systemic-violence-against-healthcare-workers-in-india.

21 Analy Nuño (2020). '"What's wrong with you Mexico?" Health workers attacked amid COVID-19 fears', *Guardian*, https://www.theguardian.com/world/2020/apr/23/mexico-health-workers-attacked-COVID-19-fears.

22 Sarah Johnson (2021). 'Spat at, abused, attacked: healthcare staff face rising violence during Covid', https://www.theguardian.com/global-development/2021/jun/07/spat-at-abused-attacked-healthcare-staff-face-rising-violence-during-covid.

23 Johnson (2021). 'Spat at, abused, attacked'.

24 BBC News (1999). 'Zero tolerance for NHS violence', http://news.bbc.co.uk/1/hi/health/473955.stm.

25 NHS England (2021). 'Chief midwife urges pregnant women to get NHS COVID jab', https://www.england.nhs.uk/2021/07/chief-midwife-urges-pregnant-women-to-get-nhs-covid-jab.

26 Professor Jacqueline Dunkley-Bent @TeamCMidO Tweet, 19 November 2021, https://twitter.com/TeamCMidO/status/1461633440105783300.

27 Megan Ford (2021). '"Enough is enough": Open letter calls for end to Covid-related abuse against health workers', *Nursing Times*, https://www.nursingtimes.net/news/coronavirus/enough-is-enough-open-letter-calls-for-end-to-covid-related-abuse-against-health-workers-04-08-2021.

28 Royal College of Midwives (2021). 'COVID – vaccines: Guidance for Pregnant women', https://www.rcm.org.uk/coronavirus-hub/covid-vaccines-for-pregnant-women/vaccine-facts; NHS England (2021). 'Chief midwife urges pregnant women to get NHS COVID jab'.

29 Megan Ford (2021). 'Union leader and NHS staff targeted
    with "vile abuse" over COVID-19 vaccines', *Nursing
    Times*, https://www.nursingtimes.net/news/coronavirus/
    union-leader-and-nhs-staff-targeted-with-vile-abuse-over-COVID-
    19-vaccines-02-08-2021.
30 Wendy Tuohy (2021). '"Eat a bat and die": Vile threats against
    Wuhan lab conspiracy-buster', *Sydney Morning Herald*, https://
    www.smh.com.au/national/eat-a-bat-and-die-vile-threats-against-
    wuhan-lab-conspiracy-buster-20210701-p5861i.html.
31 Bianca Nogrady (2021). '"I hope you die": how the COVID
    pandemic unleashed attacks on scientists', https://biancanogrady.
    com/2021/10/14/i-hope-you-die-how-the-covid-pandemic-
    unleashed-attacks-on-scientists.
32 Laura Bates (2020). *Men who hate women: from incels to pickup
    artists, the truth about extreme misogyny and how it affects us all*,
    London: Simon and Schuster.
33 Harriet Sherwood (2020). 'Midwife shortage doubles as NHS staff
    diverted to tend COVID-19 patients', *Guardian*, https://www.
    theguardian.com/society/2020/mar/29/midwife-shortage-doubles-
    as-nhs-staff-diverted-to-tend-COVID-19-patients.

8: Burnt out and Quitting

1   Emma Boyde (2019). 'Workers in Asia show high levels of physical
    and mental ill health', *Financial Times*, https://www.ft.com/
    content/cc56a824-d941-11e9-9c26-419d783e10e8.
2   Health Bureau (2017). 'Executive Summary', https://www.
    healthbureau.gov.hk/download/press_and_publications/
    otherinfo/180500_sr/e_ch1.pdf.
3   WHO (2019). 'Burn-out an "occupational phenomenon":
    International Classification of Diseases', https://www.who.int/
    news/item/28-05-2019-burn-out-an-occupational-phenomenon-
    international-classification-of-diseases.
4   WHO (2023). 'Occupational stress, burnout, and fatigue', https://
    www.who.int/tools/occupational-hazards-in-health-sector/
    occup-stress-burnout-fatigue.
5   Stefan De Hert (2020). 'Burnout in Healthcare Workers: Prevalence,
    Impact and Preventative Strategies', National Library of Medicine,
    https://www.ncbi.nlm.nih.gov/pmc/articles/PMC7604257.
6   Antonio Lasalvia et al. (2020). 'Levels of burn-out among
    healthcare workers during the COVID-19 pandemic and their
    associated factors: a cross-sectional study in a tertiary hospital of
    a highly burdened area of north-east Italy', *BMJ Open*, https://
    bmjopen.bmj.com/content/11/1/e045127.info.

7 Tom Cox, Amanda Griffiths and Sue Cox (1996). *Work-related stress in nursing: controlling the risk to health*, Geneva: ILO, https://www.ilo.org/wcmsp5/groups/public/---ed_protect/---protrav/---safework/documents/publication/wcms_250097.pdf.

8 WHO (2021). 'Protecting, safeguarding and investing in the health and care workforce', A74/A/CONF./6 Agenda Item 15, Seventy-Forth World Health Assembly, https://apps.who.int/gb/ebwha/pdf_files/WHA74/A74_ACONF6-en.pdf; WHO (2016). *Global Strategy on Human Resources for Health: Workforce 2030*, https://apps.who.int/iris/bitstream/handle/10665/250368/9789241511131-eng.pdf.

9 WHO (2022). 'WHO guideline on self-care interventions for health and well-being, 2022 revision', https://www.who.int/publications/i/item/9789240052192.

10 Jamie Smyth and Sarah Neville (2022). 'Covid, burnout and low pay: the global crisis in nursing', *Financial Times*, https://www.ft.com/content/402df6ca-5098-40ca-9cc8-bae331c39398.

11 WHO (2023). 'Occupational stress, burnout, and fatigue'; WHO/ILO (2018). *Occupational safety and health in public health emergencies: A manual for protecting health workers and responders*, https://www.ilo.org/wcmsp5/groups/public/---ed_protect/---protrav/---safework/documents/publication/wcms_633233.pdf.

12 House of Commons Health and Social Care Committee (2021). *Workforce burnout and resilience in the NHS and Social Care: Second Report of Session 2021–22*, https://committees.parliament.uk/publications/6158/documents/68766/default.

13 NHS (2020). 'We are the NHS: People Plan for 2020/21 – action for us all', https://www.england.nhs.uk/wp-content/uploads/2020/07/We-Are-The-NHS-Action-For-All-Of-Us-FINAL-March-21.pdf.

14 WHO (2016). *Global Strategy on Human Resources for Health: Workforce 2030*.

15 WHO (2022). 'WHO guideline on self-care interventions for health and well-being'.

16 Natalie Silvey (2020). https://twitter.com/silv24/status/1241447017945223169?lang=en.

17 House of Commons Health and Social Care Committee (2021). *Workforce burnout and resilience in the NHS and Social Care*.

18 Lasalvia et al. (2021). 'Levels of burn-out among healthcare workers during the COVID-19 pandemic'.

19 Dharam Kaushik (2021). 'COVID-19 and health care workers burnout: A call for global action', *Lancet* 35(100808), https://www.thelancet.com/journals/eclinm/article/PIIS2589-5370(21)00088-2/fulltext.

9: The $1 Last Mile Health Workers

1 OECD. 'Sector 1.3 Population Policies/Programmes and Reproductive Health' https://stats.oecd.org/qwids/#?x=3&y=6&f=2:262,4:1,7:2,9:85,5:4,8:85,1:1&q=2:262+4:1+7:2+9:85+5:4+8:85+1:1+3:21,22,23,24,26,27,28,29,30,31,32,33,35,36,37,38,39+6:2005,2006,2007,2008,2009,2010,2011,2012,2013,2014,2015,2016,2017,2018,2019 (accessed July 2023).
2 Community Health Worker Impact Coalition (2023). 'PROCHW Policy Dashboard', https://joinchic.org/resources/prochw-policy-dashboard.
3 Madeleine Ballard et al. (2022). 'Payment of community health workers', *Lancet Global Health* 10(9): E1242, https://www.thelancet.com/journals/langlo/article/PIIS2214-109X(22)00311-4/fulltext.
4 Christopher J. Colvin, Steve Hodgins and Henry B. Perry (2021). 'Community health workers at the dawn of a new era: 8. Incentives and remuneration', *Health Research Policy and Systems* 19 (Suppl 3): 106, https://doi.org/10.1186/s12961-021-00750-w.
5 WHO (2023). 'Community health workers density (per 10,000 population)', *Global Health Observatory/WHO*, https://www.who.int/data/gho/data/indicators/indicator-details/GHO/community-health-workers-density-(per-10-000-population).
6 Camilla Knox-Peebles (2020). 'Community health workers: the first line of defence against COVID-19 in Africa', *Bond*, https://www.bond.org.uk/news/2020/04/community-health-workers-the-first-line-of-defence-against-COVID-19-in-africa.
7 Yanan Zhang and Matthew R. Bennett (2019). 'Will I care? The likelihood of being a carer in adult life', *Carers UK* https://www.carersuk.org/media/warllcph/carersrightsdaynov19final-2.pdf.
8 Directorate of Science Technology & Innovation (2019). 'DSTI Sierra Leone's Integrated GIS Portal launched at NIDS', https://www.dsti.gov.sl/dsti-sierra-leones-integrated-gis-portal-launched-at-nids-wins-773000-grant-from-the-gates-foundation.
9 World Economic Forum (2023). 'Animated chart: Remittance flows and GDP impact by country', https://www.weforum.org/agenda/2023/01/chart-remittance-flows-impact-gdp-country.
10 Carl Baker (2023). 'Research Briefing: NHS staff from overseas: statistics', House of Commons Library, https://commonslibrary.parliament.uk/research-briefings/cbp-7783.
11 Lucina Rolewicz, Billy Palmer and Cyril Lobont (2022). 'The NHS Workforce in numbers', Nuffield Trust, https://www.nuffieldtrust.org.uk/resource/the-nhs-workforce-in-numbers.
12 Ministry of Health and Sanitation (2015). *Sierra Leone Basic*

Package of Essential Health Services 2015-2020, https://mohs2017. files.wordpress.com/2017/06/gosl_2015_basic-package-of-essential-health-services-2015-2020.pdf; Ministry of Health and Sanitation (2016). *Human Resources for Health Country Profile: Sierra Leone*, https://www.afro.who.int/sites/default/files/2017-05/ hrhprofile16.pdf.

13   WHO (2023). 'Health workforce', https://www.who.int/ health-topics/health-workforce#tab=tab_1.

14   Wilhelmina Jallah, Francis Kateh and Raj Panjabi (2018). 'Paying and investing in last-mile community health workers accelerates universal health coverage', *BMJ Opinion*, https://blogs.bmj.com/ bmj/2018/05/22/paying-and-investing-in-last-mile-community-health-workers-accelerates-universal-health-coverage.

15   Women's Budget Group (2017). 'Investing in the Care Economy', https://wbg.org.uk/analysis/investing-care-emerging-economies.

10: Women Leaders and the Most Qualified Candidate

1   Bill & Melinda Gates Foundation (2010). Press Release: 'Melinda Gates Calls for Global Action to Save Women's and Children's Lives', https://www.gatesfoundation.org/ideas/media-center/ press-releases/2010/06/melinda-gates-calls-for-global-action-to-save-womens-and-childrens-lives.

2   Global Health 50/50 (2022). 'Boards for All? A review of power, policy and people on the Boards of organisations active in global health', https://globalhealth5050.org/wp-content/themes/global-health/reports/2022/media/Boards%20for%20All_Global%20 Health%2050_50%20Report_OnlineMarch2022.pdf.

3   Sarah Hawkes et al. (2023). 'From flowers to menstrual-flow trackers: the corporatisation of women's equality and well-being', *Lancet* 402(10396) 88–90, https://www.thelancet.com/journals/ lancet/article/PIIS0140-6736(23)00456-7/fulltext.

4   This is why you should never put your current salary on a job application: not only does it diminish your value as a woman, imply you are more junior than the man you are competing with for the role (as he will probably be paid more than you), it will also enable your future employer to benchmark their pay offer against your previous pay rather than the average salary for the role. Potential employers or recruiters will ask (often repeatedly) for your current salary, but you are not obliged to tell them: just tell them how much you want to be paid.

5   Office of the President (2023). 'Africa – health: the candidate of the DRC, Dr Jean Kaseya, takes the direction of the CDC Africa', https://www.presidence.cd/actualite-detail/actualite/

afrique_sante_le_candidat_de_la_rdc_dr_jean_kaseya_prend_la_
direction_du_cdc_africa.

6   Sara Jerving (2023). 'Paul Kagame criticizes non-transparent Africa
    CDC leadership appointment', Devex, https://www.devex.com/
    news/paul-kagame-criticizes-nontransparent-africa-cdc-leadership-
    appointment-105126#.ZA-RB14mrNo.twitter.

7   Jackson Mutinda (2023). 'Bissau-Guinean doctor
    who missed Africa CDC top job cries foul', *East
    African*, https://www.theeastafrican.co.ke/tea/
    rest-of-africa/i-was-cheated-out-of-top-au-job-says-doctor-4145738.

8   Sara Jerving (2023). 'Dr Jean Kaseya is Africa CDC's new
    director general', Devex, https://www.devex.com/news/
    dr-jean-kaseya-is-africa-cdc-s-new-director-general-104985.

9   Women in Global Health (2023). 'Our members: Magda Robalo',
    https://womeningh.org/our_members/magda-robalo-md.

10 Jerving (2023). 'Paul Kagame criticizes non-transparent Africa
    CDC leadership appointment'.

11 HeForShe (2023). 'HeForShe Champions for Gender Equality',
    https://www.heforshe.org/en/champions.

12 Marie Murphy et al. (2022). 'Networking practices and gender
    inequities in academic medicine: Women's and men's perspectives',
    Lancet Clinical Medicine 45(101338), https://www.thelancet.com/
    journals/eclinm/article/PIIS2589-5370(22)00068-2/fulltext.

13 bell hooks (2013). 'Dig Deep: Beyond Lean In', *Feminist Wire*,
    https://thefeministwire.com/2013/10/17973.

11: Call (and Ignore) the Gender Expert

1   Susan A. Jones et al. (2016). '"Women and babies are dying but not
    of Ebola": the effect of the Ebola virus epidemic on the availability,
    uptake and outcomes of maternal and newborn health services
    in Sierra Leone', *BMJ Global Health* 1(3), https://gh.bmj.com/
    content/1/3/e000065.

2   UN Peacekeeping. 'Deployment and Reimbursement', https://
    peacekeeping.un.org/en/deployment-and-reimbursement (accessed
    2024).

3   Newey (2023). 'Top WHO scientist suspended amid claims of
    "misogynistic p---ing circle"'.

4   Mary E. Black (2018). '"Manels" and what to do about them',
    BMJ, https://blogs.bmj.com/bmj/files/2018/12/female-conference-
    speaker-bingo-e1348511495522.jpg.

5   Saara Särmä (2015). 'Collage: An Art-inspired
    Methodology for Studying Laughter in World
    Politics', *e-IR*, https://www.e-ir.info/2015/06/06/

collage-an-art-inspired-methodology-for-studying-laughter-in-world-politics.

12: The Power of Data

1 Michela Tindera (2016). 'Gates Foundation Pledges $80 Million To Close The Gender "Data Gap"', Women Deliver, https://womendeliver.org/press/gates-foundation-pledges-80-million-close-gender-data-gap.

2 Elizabeth Pisani (2008). *The Wisdom of Whores: Bureaucrats, Brothels, and the Business of AIDS*, London: Granta Books.

3 UNAIDS/WHO (1998). *Report on the global HIV/AIDS epidemic*, https://data.unaids.org/pub/report/1998/19981125_global_epidemic_report_en.pdf.

4 Equaldex (2023). 'Legal recognition of non-binary gender', https://www.equaldex.com/issue/non-binary-gender-recognition.

5 Sara L. M. Davis (2020). *The Uncounted: politics of data in global health*, Cambridge: Cambridge University Press.

6 Sydney Calkin (2023). *Abortion Pills Go Global: Reproductive Freedom Across Borders*, Berkeley, CA: University of California Press.

7 Adam Easton (2023). 'Polish abortion: Activist guilty of providing pills to end pregnancy', *BBC News*, https://www.bbc.co.uk/news/world-europe-64950505.

8 Serena Williams (2018). 'Serena Williams: what my life-threatening experience taught me about giving birth', *CNN*. https://edition.cnn.com/2018/02/20/opinions/protect-mother-pregnancy-williams-opinion/index.html.

9 Dorothy Roberts (1997). *Killing the Black Body: race, reproduction, and the meaning of liberty*, London: Vintage Books.

10 MBRRACE-UK (2018). *Saving Lives, Improving Mothers' Care: Lessons learned to inform maternity care from the UK and Ireland Confidential Enquiries into Maternal Deaths and Morbidity 2014–16*, https://www.npeu.ox.ac.uk/assets/downloads/mbrrace-uk/reports/MBRRACE-UK%20Maternal%20Report%202018%20-%20Web%20Version.pdf.

11 Flo (2023). 'Anonymous Mode FAQ', https://flo.health/privacy-portal/anonymous-mode-faq.

12 Alisha Haridasani Gupta and Natasha Singer (2021). 'Your App Knows You Got Your Period. Guess Who It Told?', *New York Times*, https://www.nytimes.com/2021/01/28/us/period-apps-health-technology-women-privacy.html.

13 Peter Salter (2022). 'Norfolk mother and daughter accused of illegal abortion, burning and burying body', *Lincoln Journal Star*, https://

journalstar.com/news/state-and-regional/nebraska/norfolk-mother-and-daughter-accused-of-illegal-abortion-burning-and-burying-body/article_ff99fd49-a710-5ec3-8d51-5aced3001c71.html.

14 Peter Salter (2022). 'Norfolk mother and daughter accused of illegal abortion, burning and burying body', *Lincoln Journal Star*, https://journalstar.com/news/state-and-regional/nebraska/norfolk-mother-and-daughter-accused-of-illegal-abortion-burning-and-burying-body/article_ff99fd49-a710-5ec3-8d51-5aced3001c71.html.

15 Marjery A. Beck (2023). 'Nebraska mother sentenced to 2 years in prison for giving abortion pills to pregnant daughter', *Independent*, https://www.independent.co.uk/news/ap-nebraska-norfolk-mark-johnson-republicans-b2416894.html.

16 Meta (2022). 'Correcting the Record on Meta's Involvement in Nebraska Case', https://about.fb.com/news/2022/08/meta-response-nebraska-abortion-case.

17 Johana Bhuiyan (2022). 'Facebook gave police their private data. Now, this duo face abortion charges', *Guardian*, https://www.theguardian.com/us-news/2022/aug/10/facebook-user-data-abortion-nebraska-police.

18 Hawkes et al. (2023). 'From flowers to menstrual-flow trackers'.

19 UNU-IIGH (2023). 'Re-imagining Data Governance in the context of Digital Health', https://www.youtube.com/watch?v=I-FUfuBI1VU.

20 D.I. (2019). 'The vile experiences of women in tech', *Economist*, https://www.economist.com/open-future/2019/05/03/the-vile-experiences-of-women-in-tech; Vandana Singh (2023).'The retention problem: Women are going into tech but are also driven out', *Conversation*, https://theconversation.com/the-retention-problem-women-are-going-into-tech-but-are-also-being-driven-out-200625.

21 Emily Chang (2018). *Brotopia: Breaking Up The Boys' Club of Silicon Valley*, London: Portfolio; Shanti Das (2022). 'How TikTok bombards young men with misogynistic videos', *Observer*, https://www.theguardian.com/technology/2022/aug/06/revealed-how-tiktok-bombards-young-men-with-misogynistic-videos-andrew-tate.

22 Bess Levin (2022). 'A Reminder of Just Some of the Terrible Things Elon Musk Has Said and Done', *Vanity Fair*, https://www.vanityfair.com/news/2022/04/elon-musk-twitter-terrible-things-hes-said-and-done.

Conclusion: The Driver and the Green Wave

1   The Lancet Editorial (2021). 'Miscarriage: worldwide reform of
    care is needed', *Lancet* 397(10285): 1597, https://www.thelancet.
    com/journals/lancet/article/PIIS0140-6736(21)00954-5/fulltext.
2   Sharon LaFraniere (2023). '"We're Going Away": A State's Choice
    to Forgo Medicaid Funds Is Killing Hospitals', *New York Times*,
    https://www.nytimes.com/2023/03/28/us/politics/mississippi-
    medicaid-hospitals.html.
3   Kari Paul (2020). 'Ice detainees faced medical neglect
    and hysterectomies, whistleblower alleges', *Guardian*,
    https://www.theguardian.com/us-news/2020/sep/14/
    ice-detainees-hysterectomies-medical-neglect-irwin-georgia.
4   Victoria Bekiempis (2020). 'More immigrant women say they were
    abused by Ice gynecologist', *Guardian*, https://www.theguardian.
    com/us-news/2020/dec/22/ice-gynecologist-hysterectomies-georgia.
5   UNHCR (2023). 'Operational Data Portal: Ukrainian Refugee
    Situation', https://data.unhcr.org/en/situations/ukraine.
6   Sydney Calkin (2023). *Abortion Pills Go Global: Reproductive
    Freedom across Borders,* Berkeley, CA: University of California
    Press.
7   Horacio Fernando Soria and Miguel Lo Bianco (2022). 'Thousands
    join anti-femicide march in Argentina's capital', *Reuters*, https://
    www.reuters.com/world/americas/thousands-join-anti-femicide-
    march-argentinas-capital-2022-06-04/#:~:text=According%20
    to%20the%20Women's%20Office,as%20victims%20of%20
    domestic%20violence.
8   Samantha Schmidt (2022). 'How green became the color of
    abortion rights', *Washington Post*, https://www.washingtonpost.
    com/world/interactive/2022/abortion-green-roe-wade-argentina.

Index